Lynda AOUDIA

Imaging microcrystalline arthropathies

Lynda AOUDIA

Imaging microcrystalline arthropathies

ScienciaScripts

Imprint
Any brand names and product names mentioned in this book are subject to trademark, brand or patent protection and are trademarks or registered trademarks of their respective holders. The use of brand names, product names, common names, trade names, product descriptions etc. even without a particular marking in this work is in no way to be construed to mean that such names may be regarded as unrestricted in respect of trademark and brand protection legislation and could thus be used by anyone.

Cover image: www.ingimage.com

This book is a translation from the original published under ISBN 978-620-6-70947-3.

Publisher:
Sciencia Scripts
is a trademark of
Dodo Books Indian Ocean Ltd. and OmniScriptum S.R.L publishing group

120 High Road, East Finchley, London, N2 9ED, United Kingdom
Str. Armeneasca 28/1, office 1, Chisinau MD-2012, Republic of Moldova, Europe
Printed at: see last page
ISBN: 978-620-8-08774-6

Foreword

There are three main types of microcrystalline arthropathy: gout, chondrocalcinosis and apatitic rheumatism. These pathologies frequently require further investigation by imaging. Any radiologist may be faced with the task of interpreting a standard X-ray, ultrasound, CT scan or MRI scan for diagnostic purposes, follow-up or the search for complications. These microcrystalline arthropathies require rapid diagnosis in order to efficiently guide therapeutic management and improve the patient's functional prognosis.

The aim of this book is to provide a radiological semiology of microcrystalline arthropathies for early diagnosis and, consequently, rapid management.

Prof. Lynda AOUDIA

Table of contents

Introduction

Microcrystalline arthropathies are secondary to intra-articular crystal deposits, which can trigger an intense acute inflammatory reaction or lead to chronic rheumatism. There are three main types of arthropathy:

- the drop by precipitation of sodium urate crystals;
- chondrocalcinosis due to the precipitation of calcium pyrophosphate crystals;
- apatitic rheumatism due to calcium hydroxyapatite deposits.

Considerable progress has been made in recent years in the pathophysiology and treatment of these conditions.

Imaging plays a vital role in the diagnosis of these arthropathies, as well as in their evolution, and it is essential to know how to recognize them in order to avoid diagnostic delays.

Drop

Gout, a microcrystalline arthropathy, is the osteoarticular expression of hyperuricemia, secondary to the precipitation of sodium urate crystals in the joints through excessive production and/or defective elimination of uric acid [1-6]. It is characterized by frequent episodes of acute arthritis affecting one or more joints. After several years, and in the absence of appropriate treatment, chronic tophaceous gout develops.

Gout is most often idiopathic, usually the result of a genetic abnormality causing a metabolic error, or iatrogenic, notably the use of thiazide diuretics, which should be systematically investigated [7]. It mainly affects men in their fifth decade, with a sex ratio of 20 men to one woman. In women, gout presents post-menopausally, often with a less characteristic topography and frequently sparing the feet. However, gout can occur at any age [8].

1. Imaging

Imaging plays an important role in the management of gout. Standard radiography retains its status as a routine, first-line examination. Significant progress has been made with osteoarticular ultrasound and dual-energy CT scans, introducing the ACR / EULAR 2015 (American College of Rheumatology/European League Against Rheumatism) gout classification criteria for better gout management [9].

1.1. Standard radiography

Standard radiography is the first-line examination to rule out the differential diagnoses of a gout attack and chronic uratic arthropathy [10].

The radiological signs of gout vary according to the stage of the disease.

1.1.1. Acute gout

X-ray examination is often normal [11]. Nonspecific periarticular edema or intra-articular effusion may be present.

1.1.2. Chronic gout

Radiographic signs may be delayed by 10 to 15 years after the onset of the disease [12]. It is characterized by asymmetric polyarticular disease, with a predilection for the lower limbs [13-18]. The characteristic radiological images of chronic gout correspond to the presence of one or more of the following elements [19] :

- **subcutaneous tophus**: these are masses of variable size, eccentric, asymmetrically distributed (fig. 1), dense and sometimes calcified (figs. 2, 3, 4), in some cases deforming the tips of fingers or toes (fig. 5);

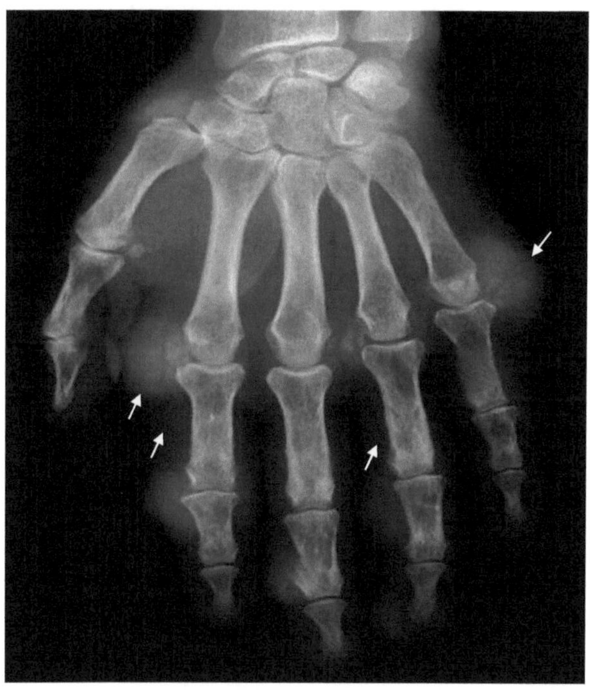

Fig. 1. Gout. Standard hand X-ray. Multiple dense, eccentric tophi (arrows).

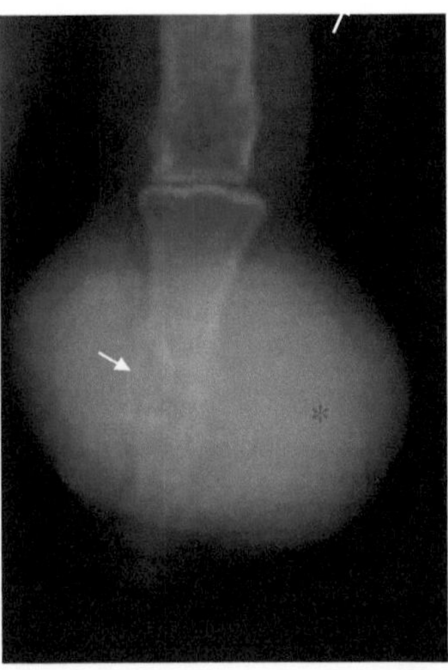

Fig. 2. Gout. Standard radiograph. Multiple dense, eccentric tophi (asterisk) associated with erosions (arrows).

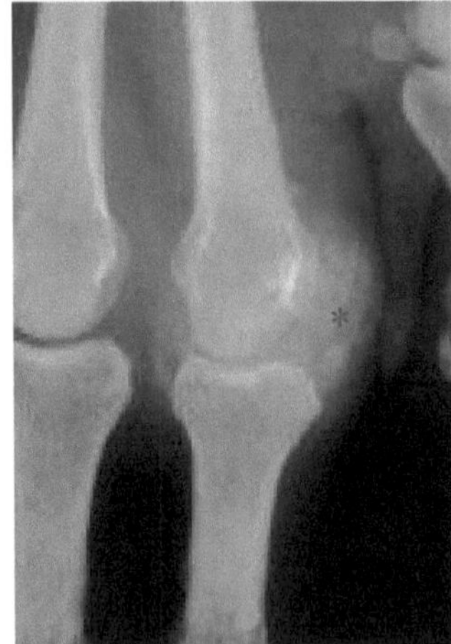

Fig. 3. Gout. Standard radiograph. Calcified Tophus (asterisk) [20].

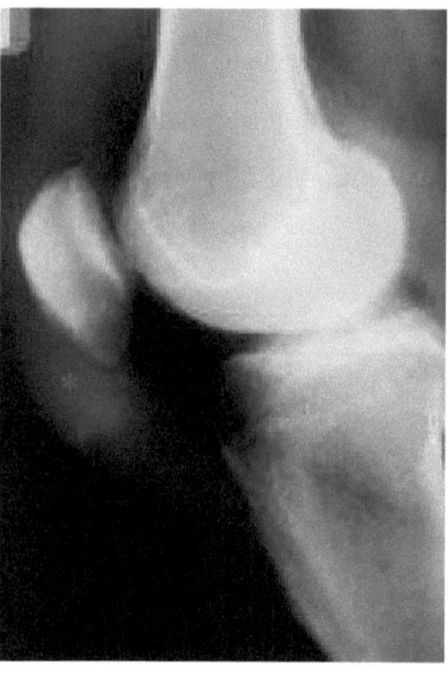

Fig. 4. Gout. Standard radiograph. Calcified prepatellar tophus (asterisk) [20].

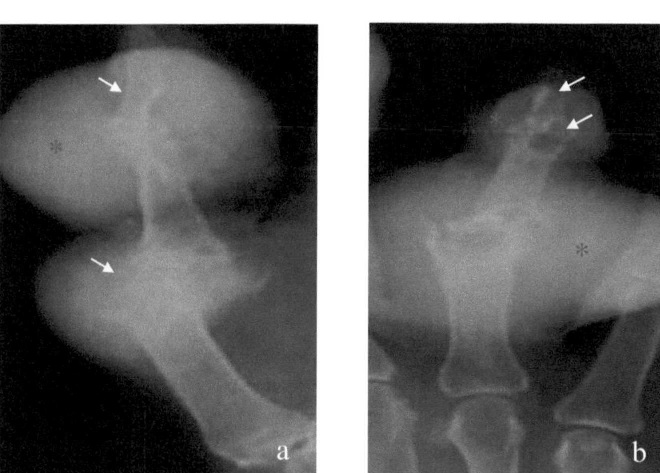

Fig. 5 Gout (a+b) Standard radiograph. Fingertip deformity (asterisk) associated with erosions (arrows).

- **eccentric para-articular bone erosions**: related to adjacent tophi. They are generally large and deep, with a long axis parallel to that of the diaphyses. They are well defined, sometimes surrounded by a condensation border (fig. 6). When they are marginal and contiguous, they produce a "halberd" appearance (fig. 7). An elevation of the erosive edge by the tophus, giving the appearance of a spicule, is highly suggestive of gout (figs. 6, 7, 8);

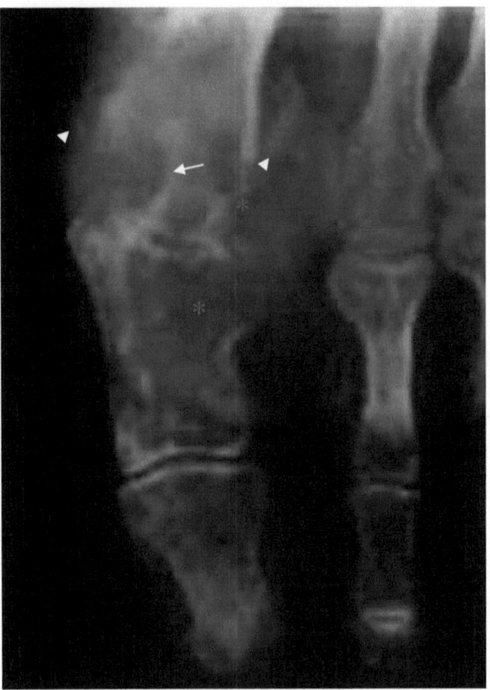

Fig. 6. Gout. Standard radiograph. Deep, asymmetrical para-articular erosions (asterisks), some surrounded by a condensation border (arrow), associated with spicules (arrowheads).

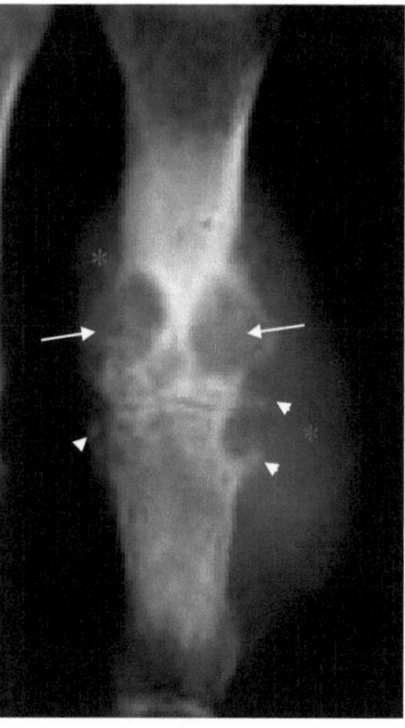

Fig. 7. Gout. Standard radiograph. Halberd-shaped erosions (arrows), associated with adjacent spicules (arrowheads) and tophi (asterisks).

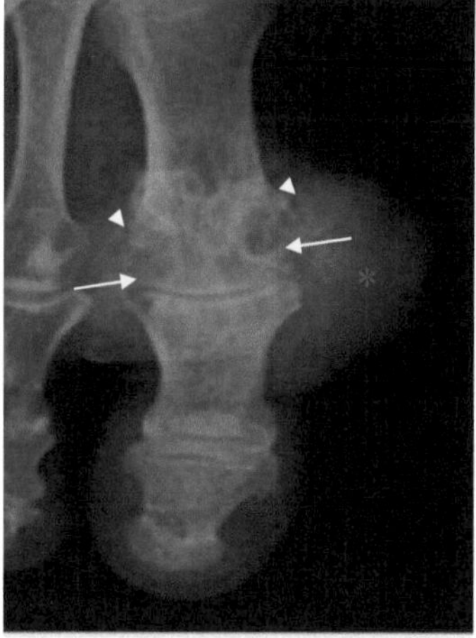

Fig. 8. Gout. Standard radiograph. Para-articular erosions (arrow), spicules (arrowheads) and adjacent tophus (asterisk).

pseudocystic intraosseous geodes: evidence of sodium urate deposits in the bone. They are rounded or oval, well-defined, cookie-cutter in shape, sometimes surrounded by a border of condensation (figs. 9, 10). They may calcify (figs. 11, 12). They vary in size, but are more than 5 mm long and parallel to the supporting bone, and are highly suggestive of gout. They may be single or multiple, centred or eccentric, but are usually located close to the joints. When they are eccentric, they thin the cortical bone and may blow out the bone (fig. 13, 14). Small, marginal geodes may mimic rheumatic arthritis (fig. 15). The presence of spicules aids diagnosis. Large geodes may destroy the joint (fig.16);

-

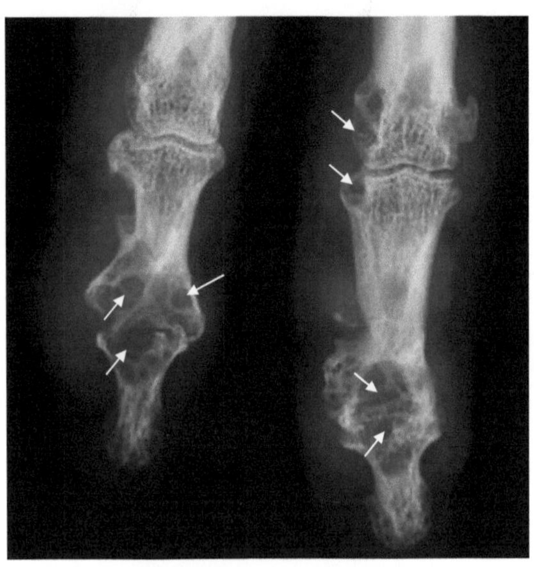

Fig. 9. Gout. Standard radiograph. Multiple intraosseous tophi (arrows).

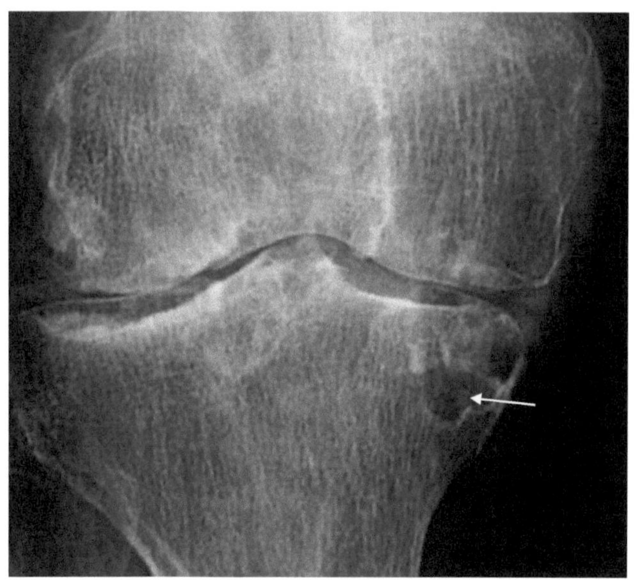

Fig. 10. Gout. Standard radiograph. Intraosseous tophus (arrow).

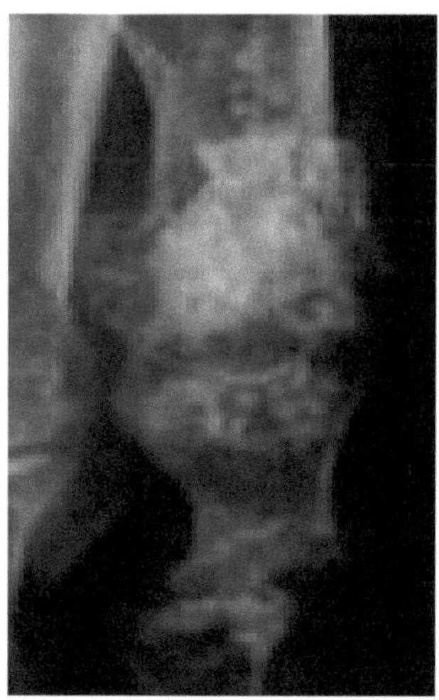

Fig. 11. Gout. Standard radiograph. Intraosseous calcified tophus (arrow).

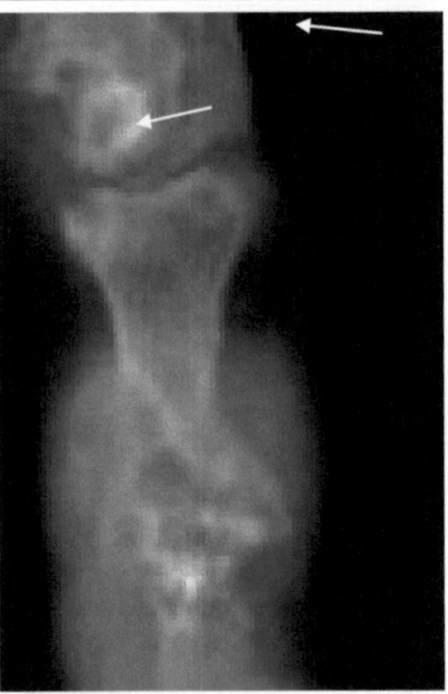

Fig. 12. Gout. Standard radiograph. Calcified intraosseous tophi (arrow), associated with non-calcified tophi [20].

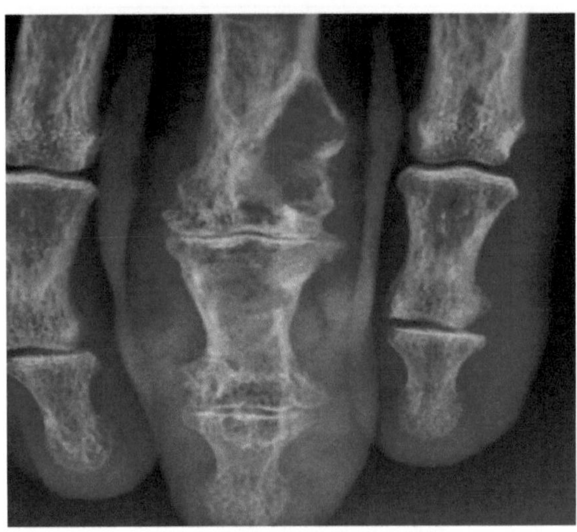

Fig. 13. Gout. Standard radiograph. Eccentric intraosseous tophus with blown cortex (arrow).

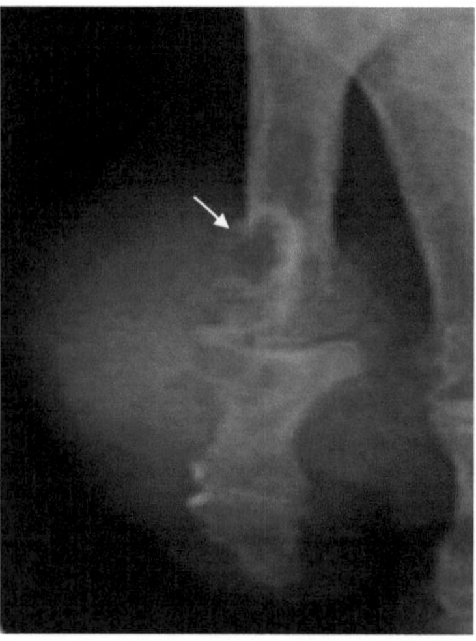

Fig. 14. Gout. Standard radiograph. Eccentric intraosseous tophus, surrounded by a border of sclerosis, blowing out the cortex (arrow).

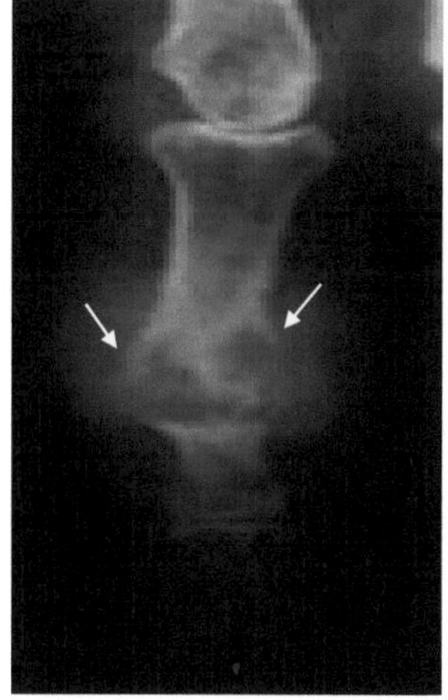

Fig. 15. Gout. Standard radiograph. Small marginal erosions, associated with diffuse joint pinching with spicules (arrows) and swelling of the soft tissues opposite.

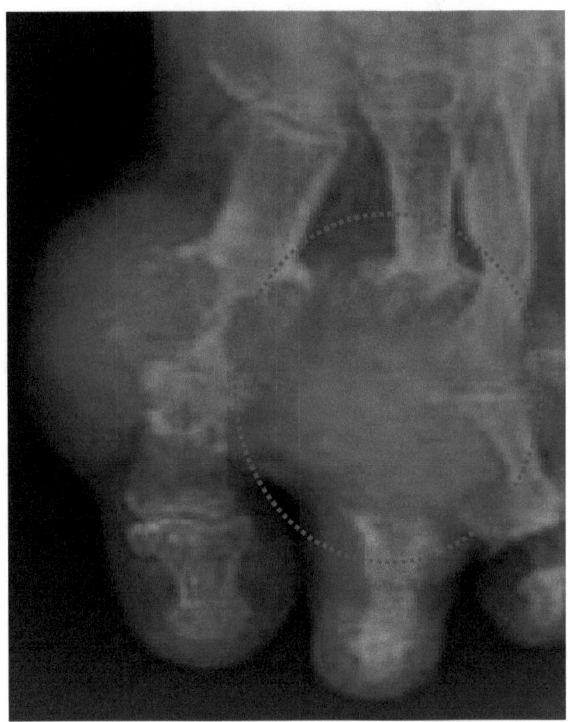

Fig. 16. Gout. Standard radiograph. Destruction of the metatarsophalangeal joint of the second radius (circle).

- **juxta-articular bone proliferations**: bone spicules reacting to the presence of adjacent tophus are sometimes exuberant, and may mimic a tumoral lesion (fig. 17); they may be periosteal appositions, voluminous osteophytes, responsible for the classic "spiky foot" (figs. 18, 19), and thick, irregular bone proliferations at tendon and muscle insertions (fig. 20);

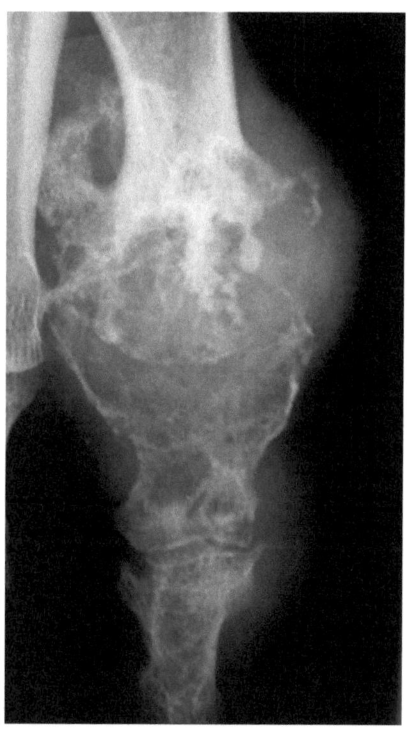

Fig. 17. Gout. Standard radiograph. Exuberant bone spicules [21].

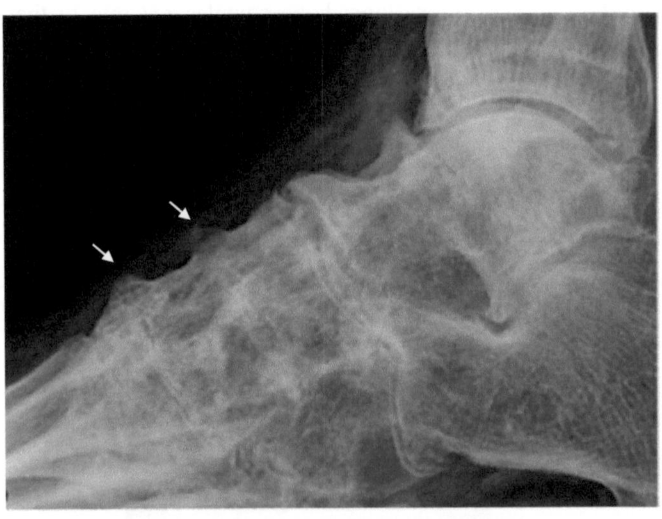

Fig. 18. Gout. Standard radiograph. Osteophytes responsible for spiky foot (arrows) [21].

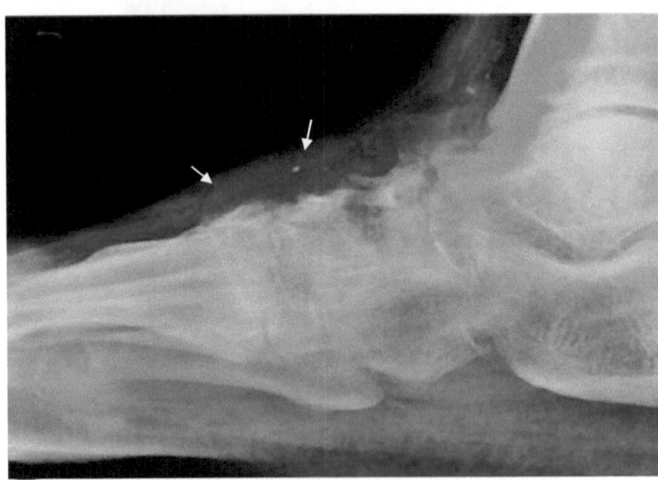

Fig. 19. Gout. Standard radiograph. Enthesophytes responsible for spiky foot (arrows) [21].

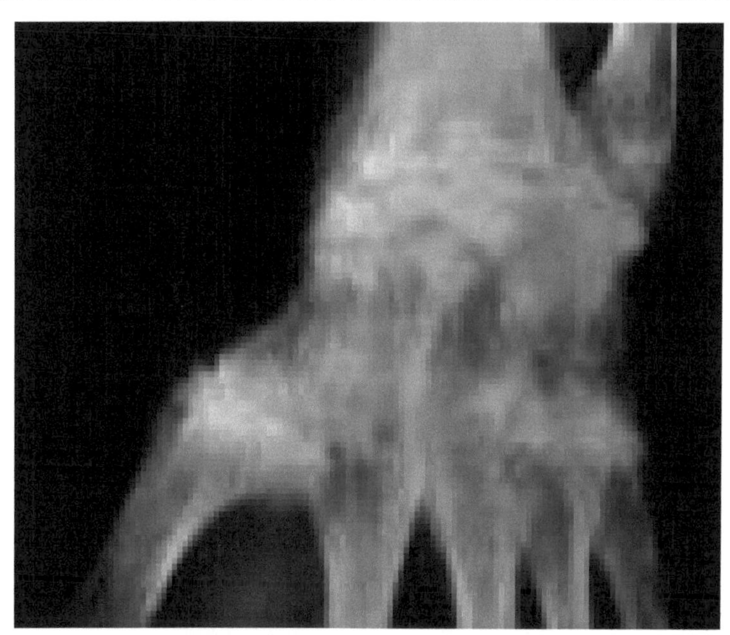

Fig. 20. Gout. Standard radiograph. Intercarpal and carpometacarpal ankylosis of gouty origin [20].

- **a long preserved joint space**, contrasting with the presence of erosions and geodes (fig. 21). Later, uniform pinching (fig. 22) and joint misalignment or destruction (fig. 23) may be observed. Bone ankylosis is rare, except in the interphalangeal joints of the hands and feet, and in the intercarpal region (fig. 20).

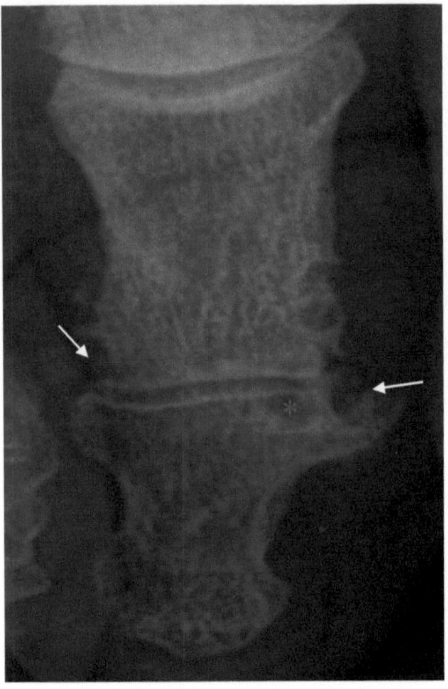

Fig. 21. Gout. Standard radiograph. Presence of erosions (arrows) and geodes (asterisk) with respected joint space.

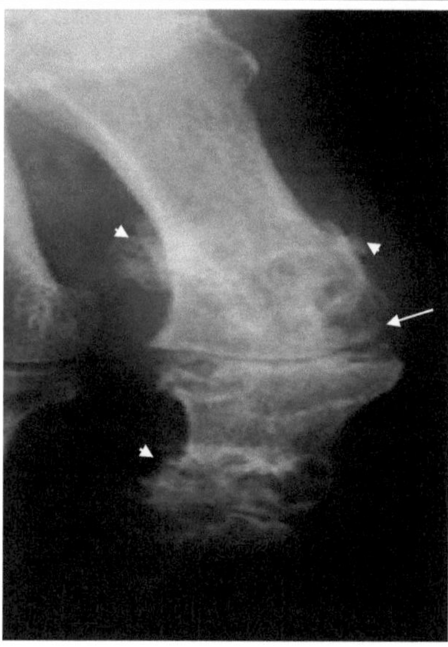

Fig. 22. Gout. Standard radiograph. Presence of erosions (arrows) and osteophytes (lip heads) with pinching of the joint space.

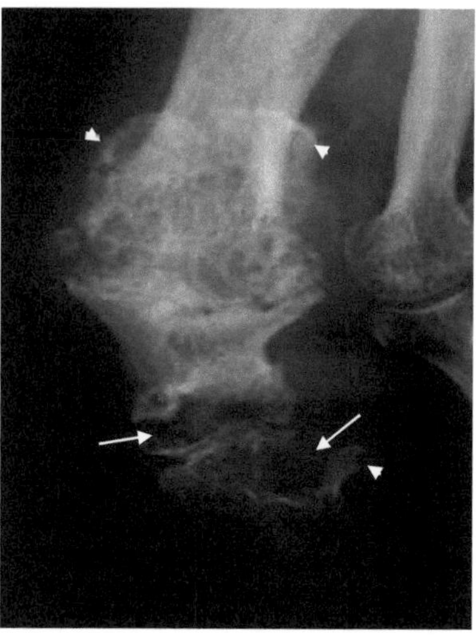

Fig. 23. Gout. Standard radiograph. Erosions (arrows), geodes (asterisk), osteophytes (arrowheads), joint destruction and misalignment.

1.1.3. Radiological signs according to lesion location

1.1.3.1.Feet

Involvement of the metatarsophalangeal joints is the most common:

- **Early stage**

- Erosions often present as a simple irregularity of the cortical surface of the medial and dorsal faces of the first metatarsal head [17] (fig. 24) ;
- soft tissue swelling adjacent to erosions;
- widening and irregularity of the first metatarsal head (fig. 25);
- hallux-valgus bone deformities are often associated;

- **Late stage**

- Erosions and open geodes in the joint can lead to complete osteolysis of the head of the first metatarsal.
- marked pinching of the joint line, even ankylosis;
- involvement of other metatarsophalangeal joints, particularly of the fifth radius and interphalangeal joints [22] (fig. 26);
- involvement of the hindfoot mainly concerns the mediotarsal joints, with dorsal osteophytes of the talonavicular and naviculocuneal joints giving a "spiky foot" appearance (figs. 18, 19), and retro- and subcalcaneal bony outgrowths. A voluminous tophus is sometimes responsible for the destruction of several tarsal bones (fig. 27);
- ankle involvement is rare, presenting as malleolar geodes and marginal osteophytes (fig. 28).

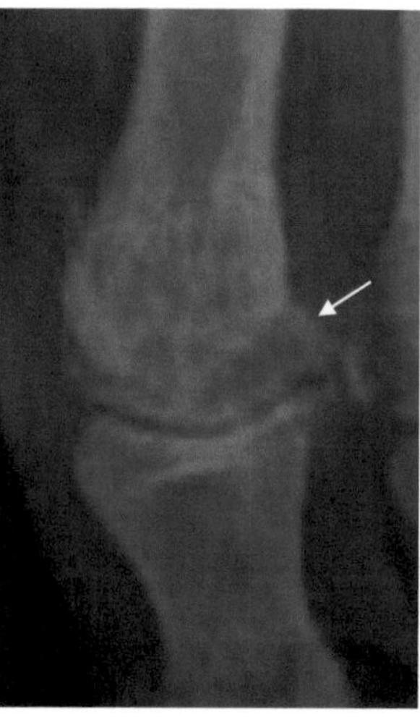

Fig. 24. Gout. Standard radiograph. Irregularities on the medial surface of the first metatarsal head (arrow).

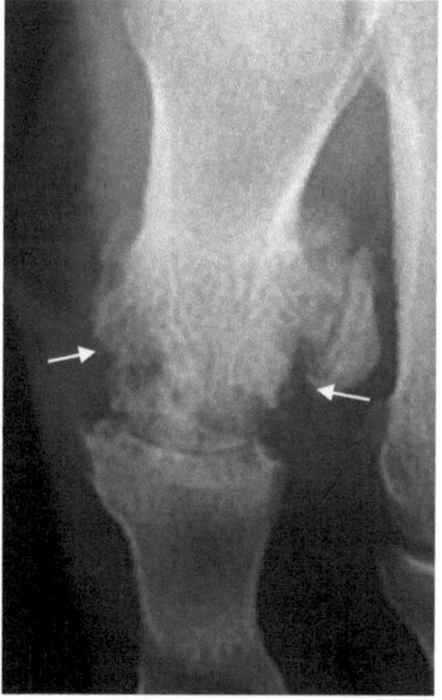

Fig. 25. Gout. Standard radiograph. Enlargement and irregularity of the first metatarsal head (arrows).

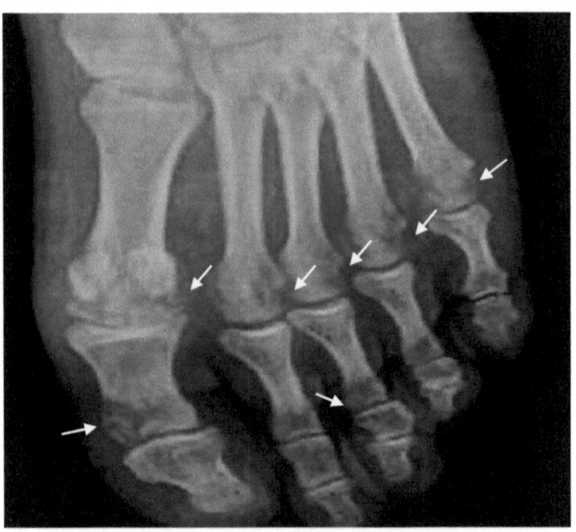

Fig. 26. Gout. Standard radiograph. Erosions of the metatarsophalangeal and interphalangeal heads (arrows).

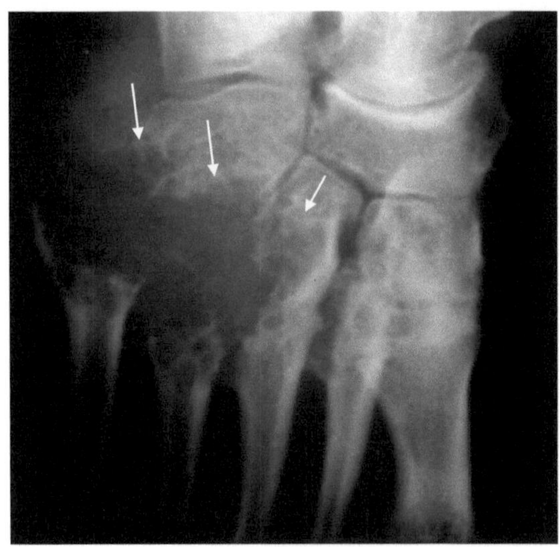

Fig. 27. Gout. Standard radiograph. A voluminous tophus responsible for the destruction of several tarsal bones (arrows).

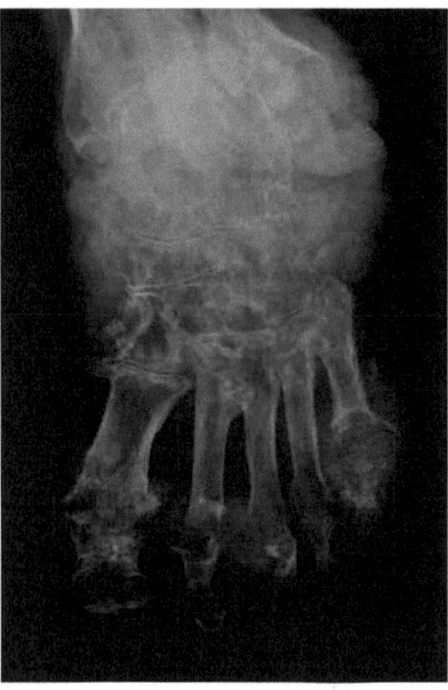

Fig. 28. Gout. Standard radiograph. Multiple tophi, erosions and osteophytes on the foot and ankle.

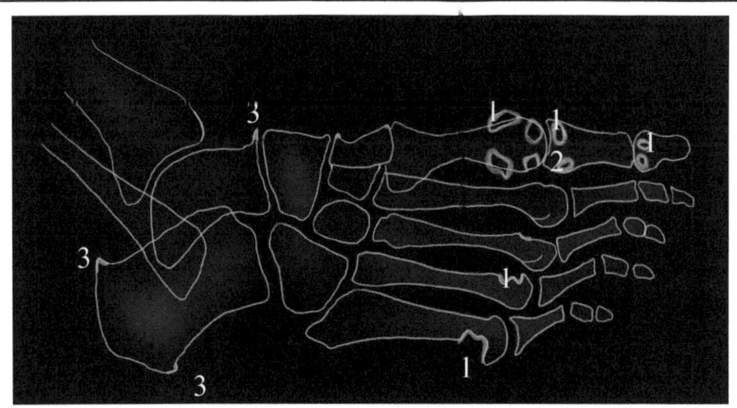

Fig. 29. Gout. Foot involvement. Diagram. (1) Bone erosions and geodes with intraosseous tophi; (2) gouty arthropathy of the big toe with joint pinching; (3) intertarsal and calcaneal gouty arthropathy with sharp tophi and "spiky foot" image.

1.1.3.2.Hands and wrists

- involvement of the interphalangeal joints and, to a lesser degree, the metacarpophalangeal joints (figs. 1, 2, 3, 5, 6, 7, 9, 12, 13, 17, 30);
- erosions of the carpus and carpometacarpal joints (fig. 31);
- a voluminous tophus destroys the carpal bones, mainly the ulnar margin.

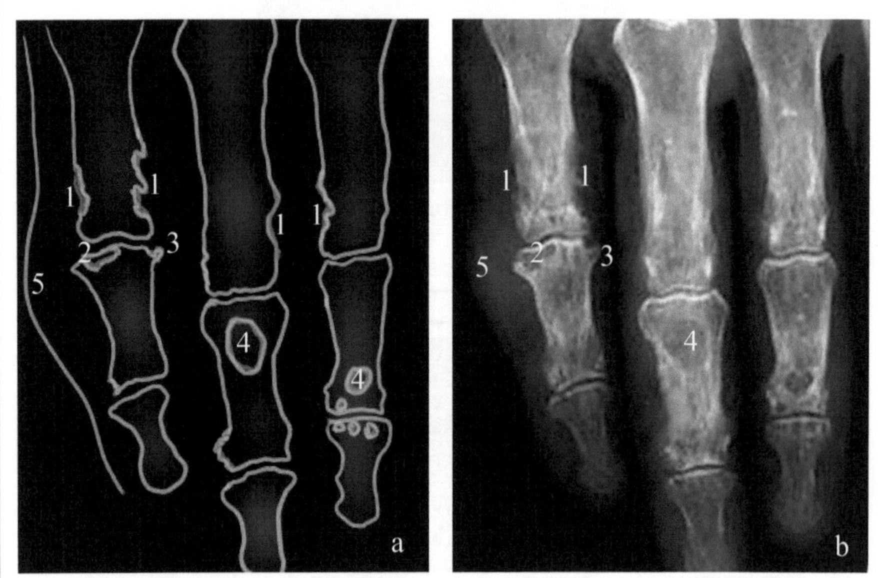

Fig. 30. Gout. (a) Diagrams. (b) Standard radiograph. (1) Cortical irregularity. (2) Erosions. (3) Osteophytes. (4) Intraosseous geodes. (5) Tophus responsible for soft-tissue swelling.

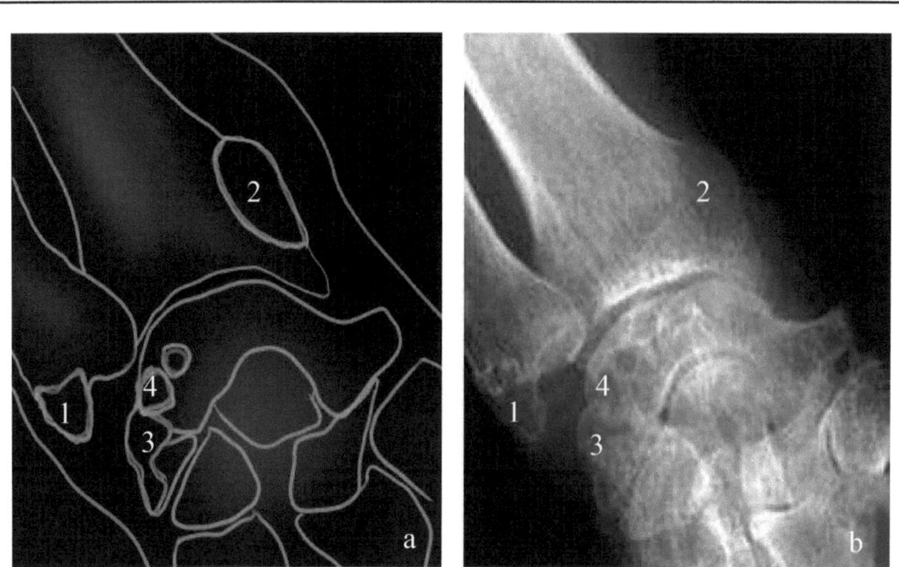

Fig. 31. Gout. (a) Schematic diagrams. (b) Standard radiograph. (1) Erosion of the lower end of the ulna**.** (2) Erosion of the lower end of the radius. (3) Erosion of the triquetrum. (4) Semilunar geodes.

1.1.3.3.Knee

- Notches on the lateral and medial surfaces of the tibial plateaus and femoral condyles (fig. 32);
- femoral or tibial intraosseous geodes (fig. 10) [23, 24] ;
- involvement of the patella by the presence of finely encircled erosions with bone spicules reacting to prepatellar tophus (fig. 33, 34).

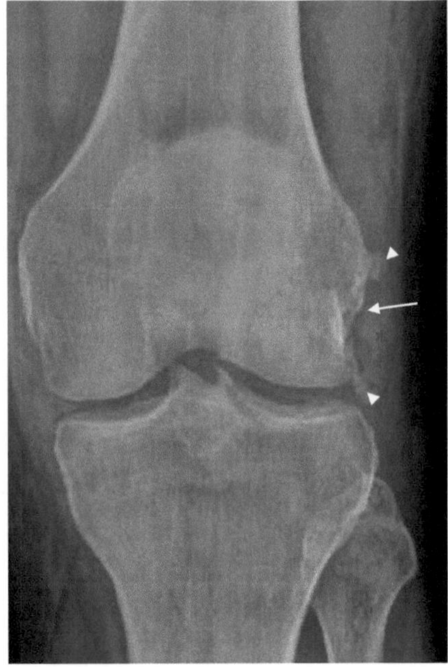

Fig. 32. Gout. Involvement of the knee. Standard radiograph. Erosion of lateral aspect of femoral condyle (arrow), osteophytes (arrowheads) and tophus (asterisk) opposite.

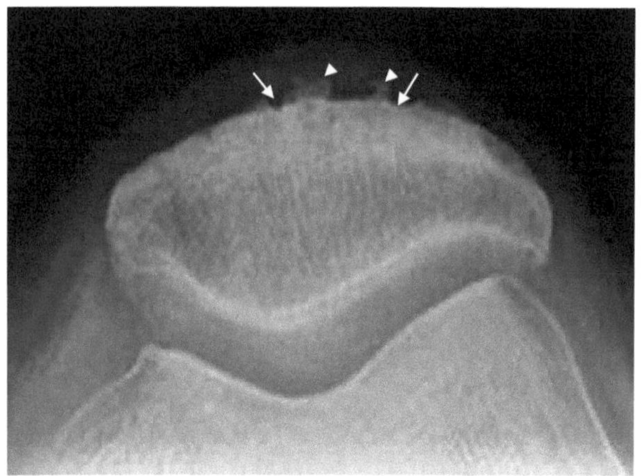

Fig. 33. Gout. Involvement of the knee. Standard radiograph. Erosions of the anterior aspect of the patella (arrows), associated with prepatellar bone constructions (arrowheads).

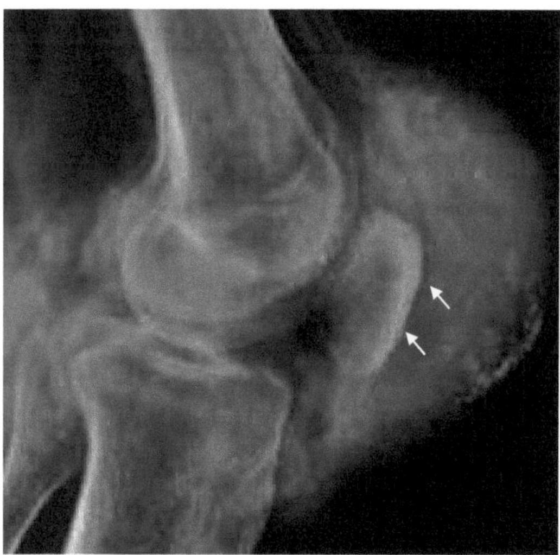

Fig. 34. Gout. Involvement of the knee. Standard radiograph. Tophus opposite the patella (asterisk) with irregularity of the cortical surface of the anterior aspect of the patella (arrow).

1.1.3.4.Elbow

bursitis on the dorsal surface of the olecranon, associated with bone erosions and proliferations (figs. 35, 36).

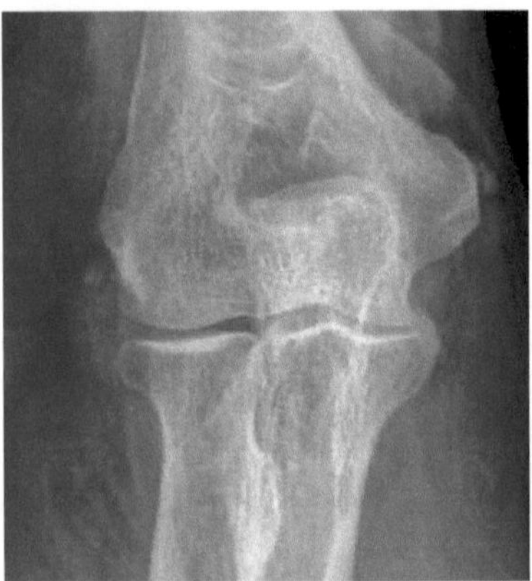

Fig. 35. Gout. Elbow involvement. Standard radiograph. Tophus of elbow (asterisk).

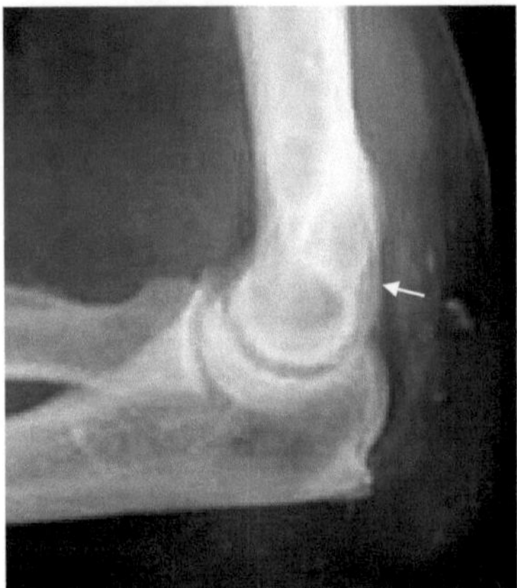

Fig. 36. Gout. Elbow involvement. Standard radiograph. Irregularity of the posterior surface of the lower end of the humerus (arrow) and calcified tophus opposite (asterisk).

1.1.3.5.Other joints

- Involvement of the shoulder and hip is rare, presenting as soft tissue swelling, bone erosions, pseudocystic lesions and/or bone proliferation (fig. 37).
- Sacroiliac joints are characterized by an irregular, scalloped appearance of the joint margins (fig. 38).
- In the spine, involvement is manifested by erosions of the odontoid, vertebral endplates and zygapophyseal joints, disc pinches and vertebral subluxations [24-31]. Occasionally, spinal cord compression secondary to the presence of extradural deposits of sodium urate crystals;
- extremely rare involvement of the temporomandibular, cricoarytenoid, costochondral and manubriosternal joints.

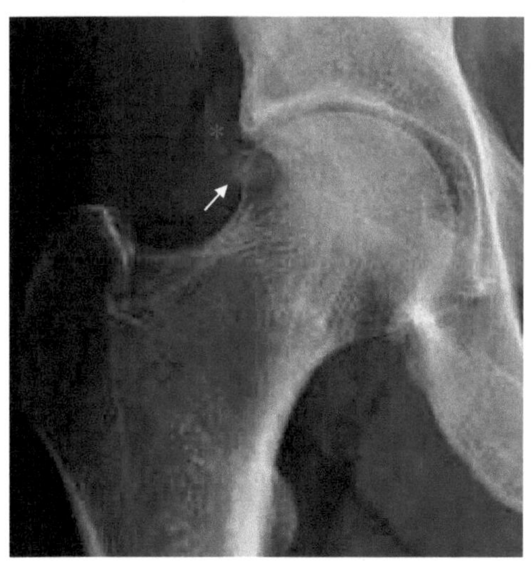

Fig. 37. Gout. Hip involvement. Standard radiograph. Bone proliferation (arrow) and opposing tophus (asterisk).

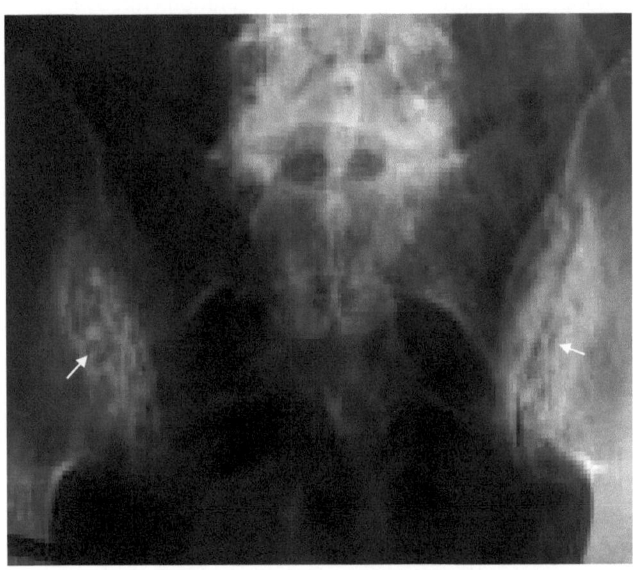

Fig. 38. Gout. Sacroiliac involvement. Standard radiograph. Bilateral, well-limited sacroiliac erosions bordered by osteocondensation (arrows) [20].

1.2. Ultrasound

Osteoarticular ultrasound enables the diagnosis and follow-up of gouty arthropathy. It is used in the 2015 ACR/EULAR gout classification criteria [9].

1.2.1. Non-specific ultrasound signs of gout

As with any potentially destructive rheumatism, certain signs may be found without being specific to gout [32-34]. OMERACT (International Outcome Measures in Rheumatology Clinical Trials) has developed definitions of common ultrasound signs of inflammatory arthritis [35] :

- **Joint effusion**: abnormal, hypo- or anechogenic intra-articular material, in comparison with subcutaneous fat, partially compressible with the probe but without Doppler signal (fig. 39). This material may be rarely iso or even hyperechoic. The presence of hyperechoic spots in the fluid suggests a microcrystalline pathology, but is not specific to gout.
- **Synovitis**: Abnormal intra-articular structure, hypoechoic in relation to subcutaneous fat, non-dispersible and poorly compressible with a probe, may be vascularized by Doppler. This structure may rarely be iso or hyperechoic. The presence of hyperechoic spots in the synovium is highly suggestive in the clinical context of gout [36].
- **Tenosynovitis**: Hypo or anechoic thickening, with or without fluid, located within the tenosynovial sheath, which can be objectified in two planes of section (fig. 40). This structure may or may not contain a Doppler signal.
- **Erosion**: Intra- and/or extra-articular discontinuity of the bone surface, visible in two perpendicular planes.

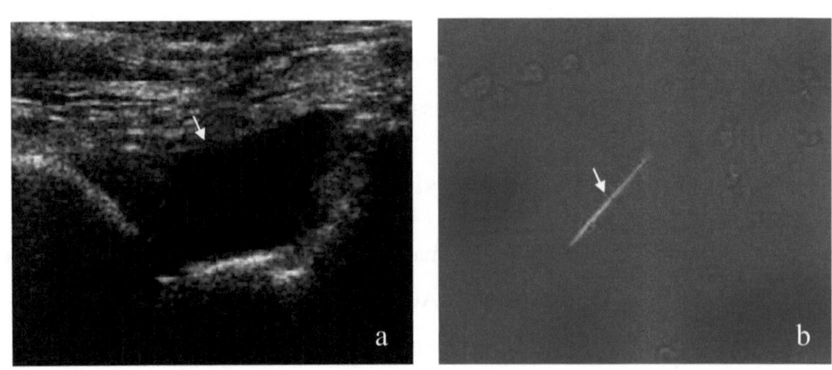

Fig. 39. Gout (a) Ultrasound. Joint effusion, anechoic (arrow). (b) Microscopy of synovial fluid. Monosodium urate crystals under compensated polarizing light microscopy [37].

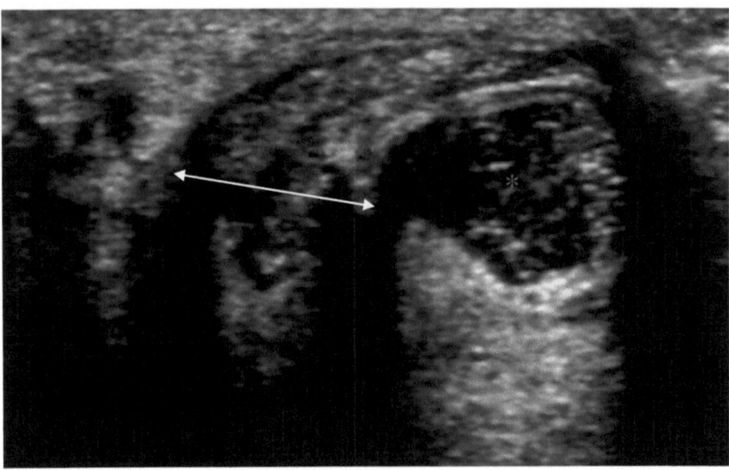

Fig. 40. Gout. Ultrasound. Hypoechoic tenosynovial thickening (bidirectional arrow) and tophus (asterisk).

1.2.1.1.Specific ultrasound signs of gout

Certain signs are highly suggestive of gout [38, 39]. OMERACT has defined four basic ultrasound signs of gout [40, 41].

- **Double contour**: Abnormal hyperechoic band on the superficial edge of the cartilage, independent of the probe angle. The band may be irregular or regular, continuous or intermittent. Distinguishable from cartilage interface sign (figs. 41, 42, 43).

- **Tophus**: circumscribed, inhomogeneous, hyperechoic and/or hypoechoic aggregation with or without a posterior acoustic shadow cone, which may be surrounded by a small anechogenic halo. Location may be intra-articular, extra-articular or intra-tendinous (figs. 44, 45, 46, 47).

- **Aggregates**: Heterogeneous hyperechogenic foci that retain their high degree of reflectivity even when the gain setting is minimized or the probe angle is changed, sometimes with a posterior acoustic shadow cone, giving a "snowstorm" appearance (fig. 48).

- **Erosion**: intra- and/or extra-articular discontinuity of the bone surface, visible in two perpendicular planes (fig. 49).

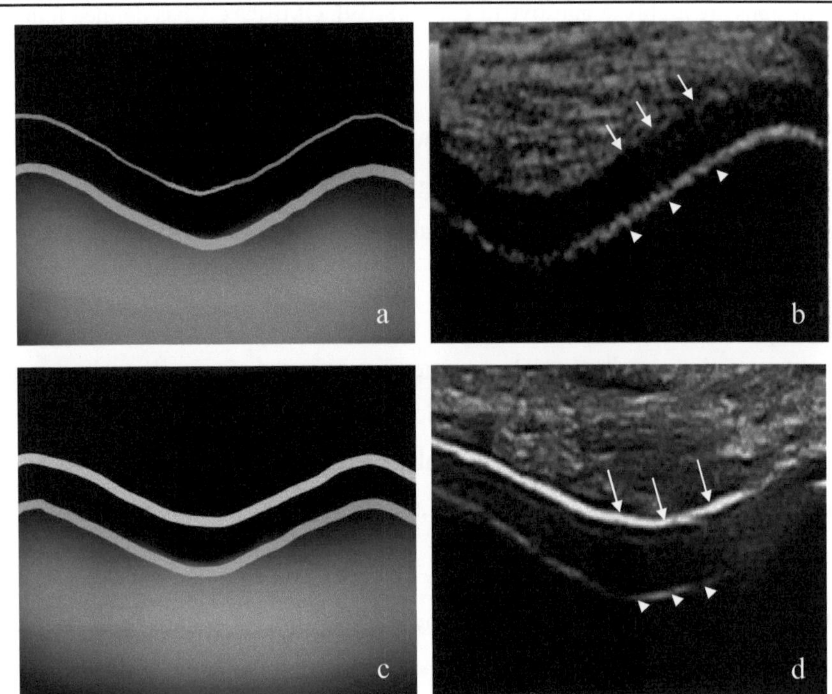

Fig. 41. Gout (a+c) Diagrams. (b+d) Ultrasound sections. (a+b). Normal anechogenic cartilage surface (arrows), cortical bone (arrowheads). (c+d) Continuous hyperechoic band on cartilage surface (arrows), giving appearance of double contour of bone (arrowheads).

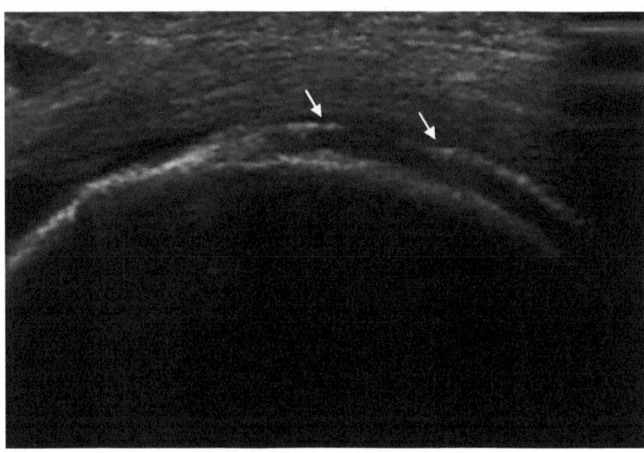

Fig. 42. Gout. Ultrasound section. the appearance of a double discontinuous contour (arrows) [42].

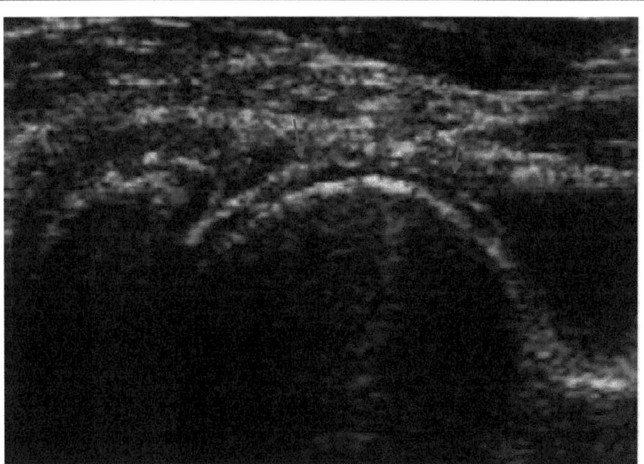

Fig. 43. Gout. Ultrasound section. double irregular contour (arrows) [37].

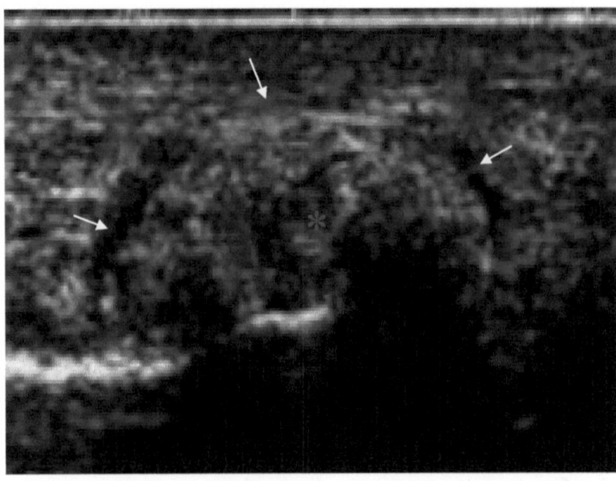

Fig. 44. Drop. Tophus. Longitudinal ultrasound section of the dorsal aspect of the metatarsophalangeal joint. Isoechogenic mass (asterisk) with posterior attenuation and surrounded by a hypoechoic halo (arrows) [43].

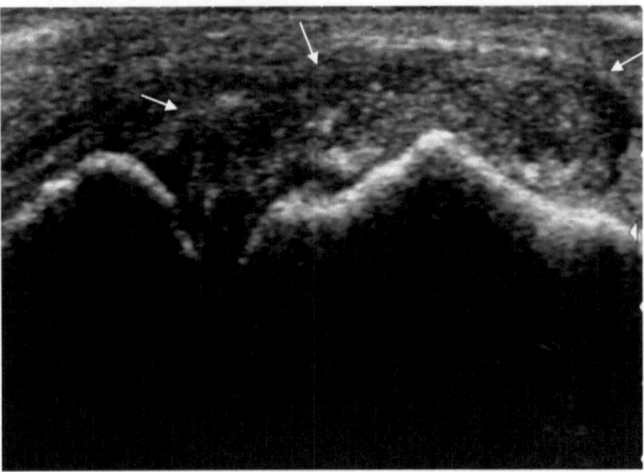

Fig. 45. Drop. Tophus. Longitudinal ultrasound section of the dorsal surface of the distal interphalangeal joint. Intra-articular tophus (asterisk) surrounded by a hypoechoic halo (arrows).

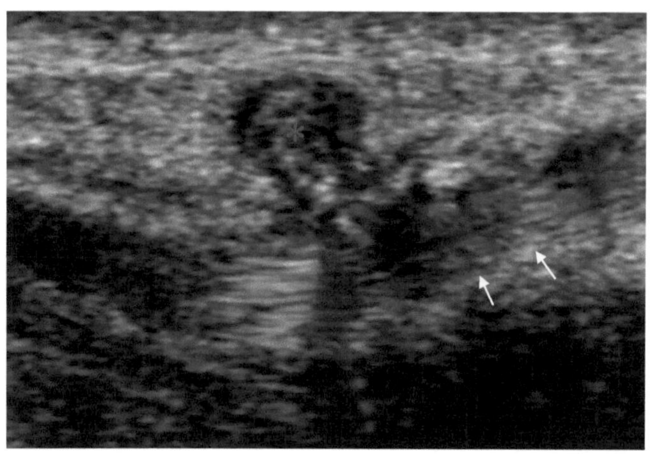

Fig. 46. Drop. Tophus. Ultrasound section. Peri-tendinous tophus (asterisk). Tendon (arrows).

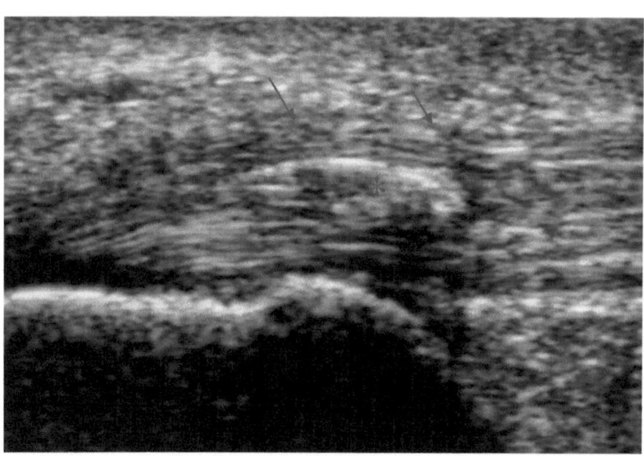

Fig. 47. Drop. Tophus. Ultrasound section. Intratendinous tophus (asterisk).

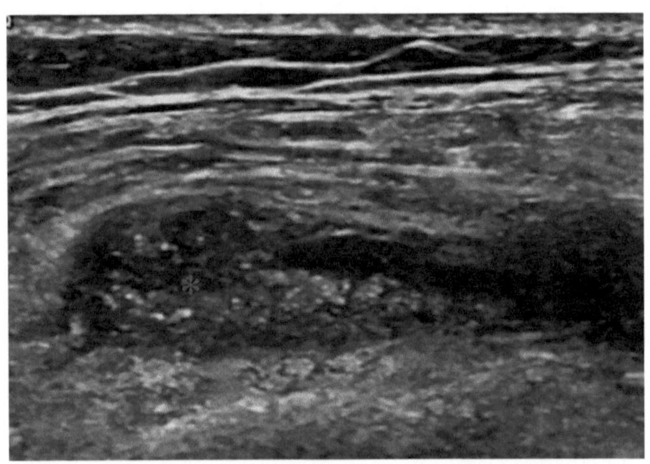

Fig. 48. Drop. Aggregates of urate crystals. Ultrasound section. Joint effusion with snowstorm appearance (asterisk) [44].

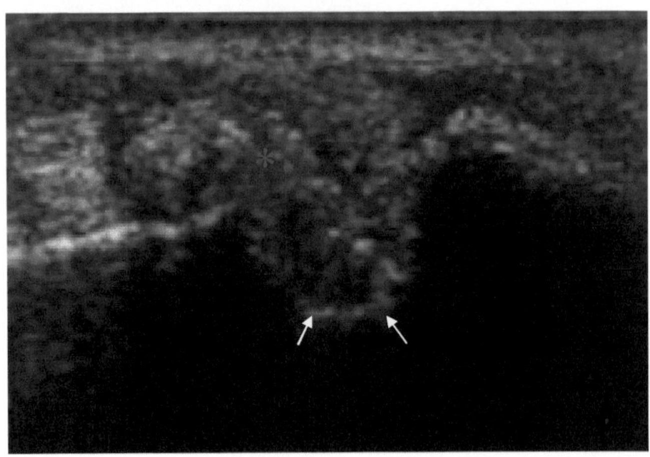

Fig. 49. Drip. Erosion. Longitudinal metatarsophalangeal ultrasound section: erosion (arrows) secondary to isoechoic tophus (asterisk) [45].

1.3. Dual-energy spectral scanner

The dual-energy spectral scanner (DECT) is a new CT imaging technique that differentiates deposits according to their different X-ray spectra. It applies the concept of tissue attenuation according to density, atomic number and photon beam energy [46].

DECT can locate and quantify monosodium urate crystal deposits in joints, ligaments, tendons and soft tissues [47] (fig. 50). This examination is included in the 2015 ACR/EULAR gout classification criteria [9]. On the other hand, this technique cannot assess inflammation or detect low-density tophus or tophus smaller than 2 mm in size [48, 49].

DECT is rarely used in current practice, due to the unavailability of equipment, its high cost and the high level of radiation involved [50].

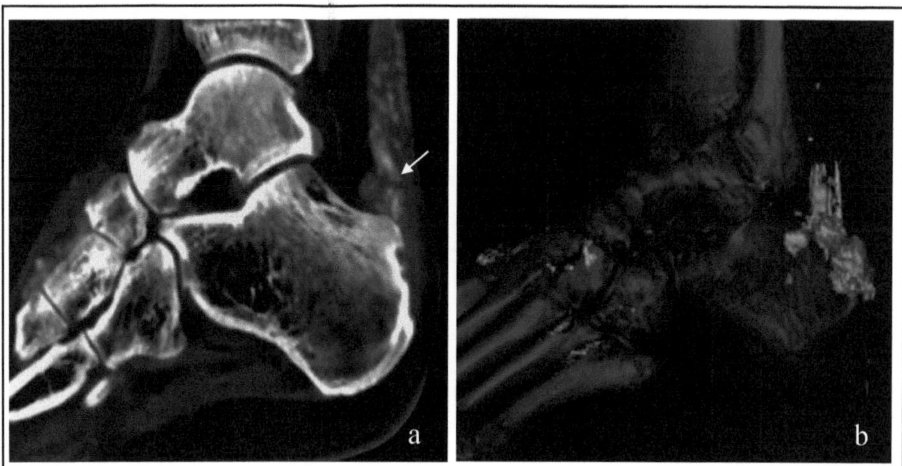

Fig. 50. Gout (a) CT scan of the foot, sagittal reconstruction. Thickening of the Achilles tendon with calcifications within it (arrow). (b) DECT. DECT of the foot showing massive green-coded tophaceous deposits [51].

1.4. MRI

The tophus presents as a homogeneous T1 hyposignal and a heterogeneous T2 hyposignal, depending on the degree of hydration [52] (fig. 51). MRI may show synovial thickening, effusion, erosions and bone edema.

The diagnostic performance of MRI for gout has not been clearly established due to the non-specific nature of the findings. MRI has therefore not been included in the ACR / EULAR gout classification criteria.

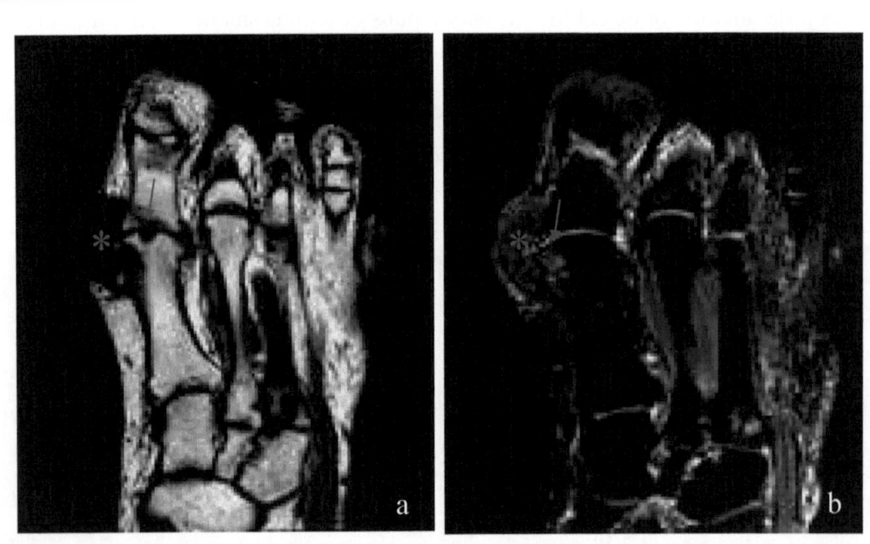

Fig. 51. Gout. MRI of the foot in axial slices (a) T1-weighted sequence. (b) T2-weighted sequence. Tophus level of the 1st metatarsophalangeal joint in T1 and T2 hyposignal (asterisk) and erosions (arrows) [51].

Joint chondrocalcinosis

Chondrocalcinosis is a joint disorder characterized by the accumulation of calcium pyrophosphate crystals in the joints, which can cause pain, inflammation and cartilage damage. It may be isolated or associated with other metabolic diseases, such as hemochromatosis, hypomagnesemia, hyperparathyroidism, familial hypercalcemia-hypocalciuria and hypophosphatasia [53]. It affects women slightly more than men, and the number of people affected increases with age [54-56]. It sometimes presents as a pseudoarthritic picture, mimicking degenerative joint damage, which is generally bilateral and symmetrical. It may also present as pseudogout, acute arthritis with significant inflammatory signs.

rapidly destructive arthropathy mimicking nervous osteoarthropathy [57, 58]; pseudorhumatoid arthritis with morning rash and synovial swelling [58].

1. Imaging

1.1. Standard radiography

1.1.1. Basic radiological signs

Involvement is often bilateral and generally symmetrical:

- intra-articular calcifications, in the form of a fine, more or less extensive opaque border, encircling the articular contours a few millimetres from the subchondral bone and showing classic cartilage encrustation (fig. 52) ;
- discontinuous calcification of the fibrocartilage of the symphysis pubis, knee menisci, intervertebral discs and carpal triangular ligaments (fig. 53, 54);
- calcifications of synovial tissue, tendons, ligaments and joint capsules, mainly in the knees.

In advanced forms, joint damage with joint destruction due to the presence of bone erosions, subchondral geodes, osteolysis and bone production in the form of subchondral osteosclerosis and osteophytosis.

The diagnosis of chondrocalcinosis should be considered whenever a joint usually spared from arthrosis is affected by degenerative phenomena, such as the atloido-axoid and metacarpo-phalangeal joints of the 2eme and 3eme fingers.

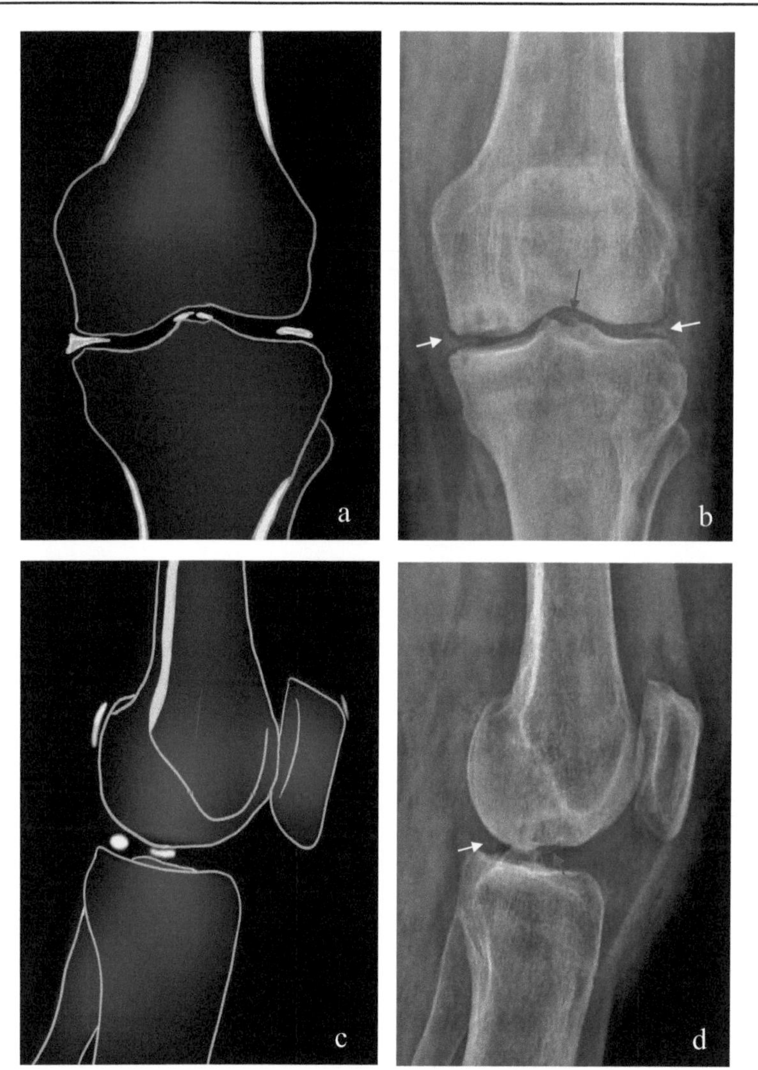

Fig. 52. Articular chondrocalcinosis. (a+c) Diagrams. (b+d) X-ray of knee, front and side. Meniscal calcifications (white arrows) and intracartilaginous opaque border (red arrows).

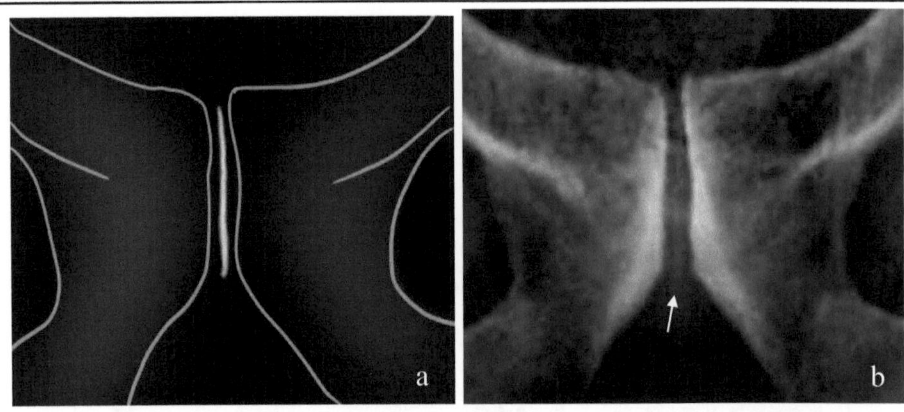

Fig. 53. Articular chondrocalcinosis. (a) Diagrams. (b) Frontal radiograph of the pubic symphysis. Intracartilaginous opaque border of the pubic symphysis (arrows).

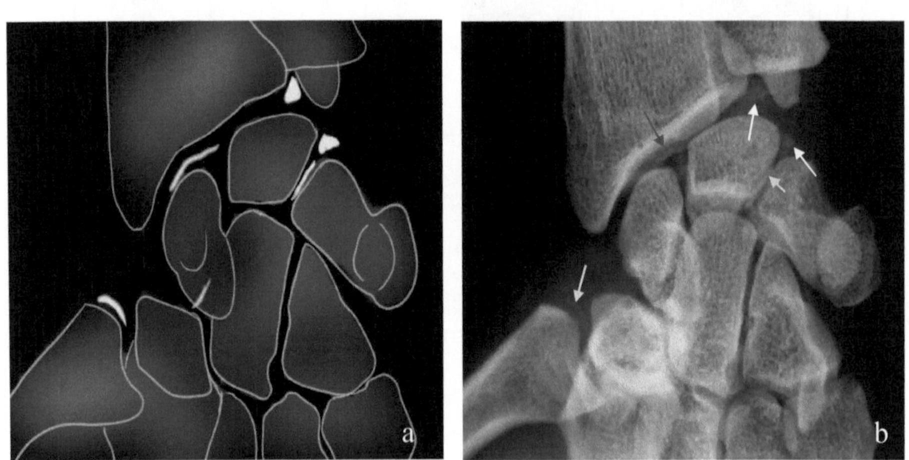

Fig. 54. Articular chondrocalcinosis. (a) Diagrams. (b) Front X-ray of the hand. Calcifications of the carpal triangular ligament (white arrow), hyaline cartilage (yellow arrows) and scapholunate and lunotriquetral ligaments (red arrow).

1.1.2. Radiological signs according to lesion location

1.1.2.1.Knees

The most common location for chondrocalcinosis. Deposits usually involve the cartilage, menisci and tendons of the twins [59, 60] (figs. 55, 56, 57, 58). These calcifications are faint, fine and linear. Destructive lesions can be seen in chronic arthropathy by the presence :

- abrasion of patellar cartilage (fig. 59);
- appearance of subchondral bone geodes (fig. 60);
- notches on the anterior surface of the femoral metaphyses in the supra-rotary region (figs. 59, 61);
- alteration of the tibial plateaus and condyles, with possible misalignment (fig. 62);
- supratrochlear erosions ;
- pseudoarthritic images with total pinching of the joint space and a thin layer of subchondral osteosclerosis on either side of the joint, giving a rail-like image (fig. 63).

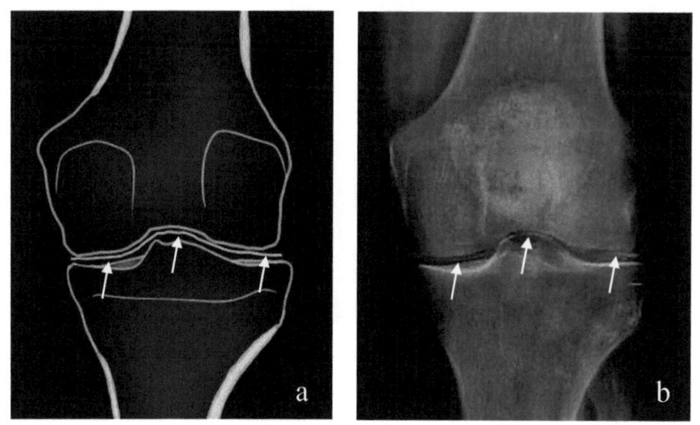

Fig. 55. Articular chondrocalcinosis. (a) Diagrams. (b) Frontal radiograph of knee. Calcifications of hyaline cartilage (arrows).

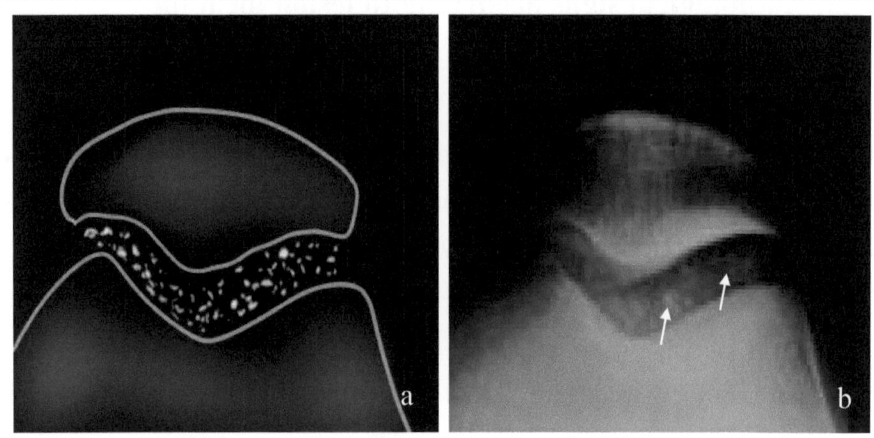

Fig. 56. Articular chondrocalcinosis. (a) Diagrams. (b) X-ray of the patellofemoral groove. Granular calcifications of the patellofemoral cartilage (arrows) [61].

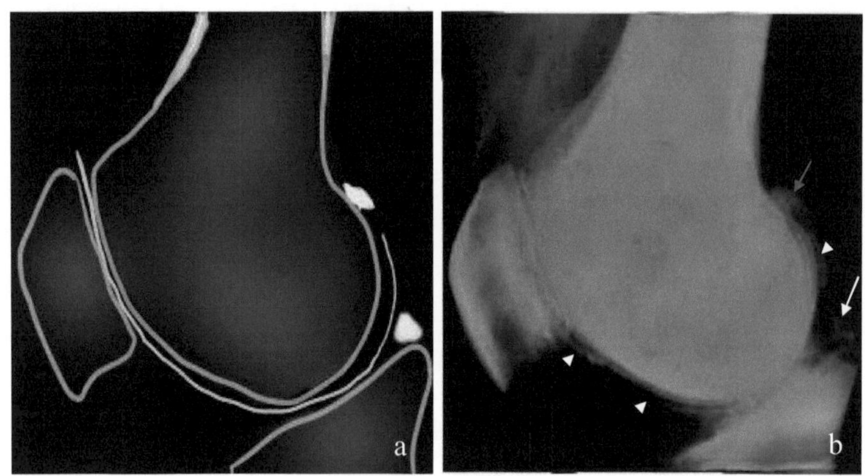

Fig. 57. Articular chondrocalcinosis. (a) Diagrams. (b) Profile X-ray of knee. Calcifications of hyaline cartilage (arrowheads), meniscal calcification (white arrow) and calcifications of gastrocnemius tendons (red arrow).

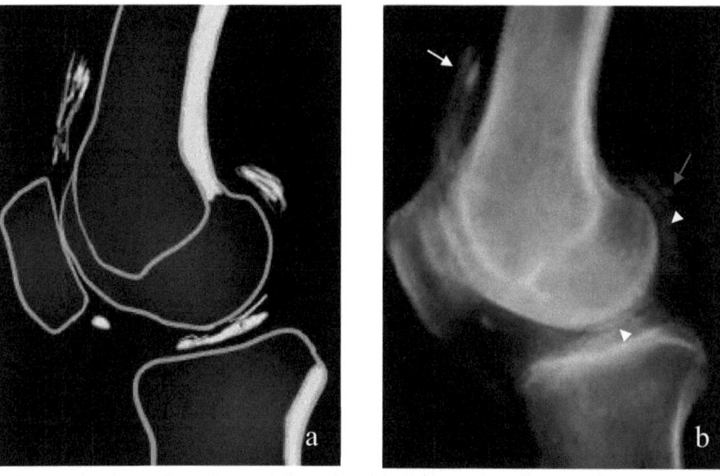

Fig. 58. Articular chondrocalcinosis. (a) Diagrams. (b) Profile X-ray of knee. Calcifications of hyaline cartilage (arrowheads), calcifications of quadriceps tendons (white arrow) and calcifications of gastrocnemius tendons (red arrow).

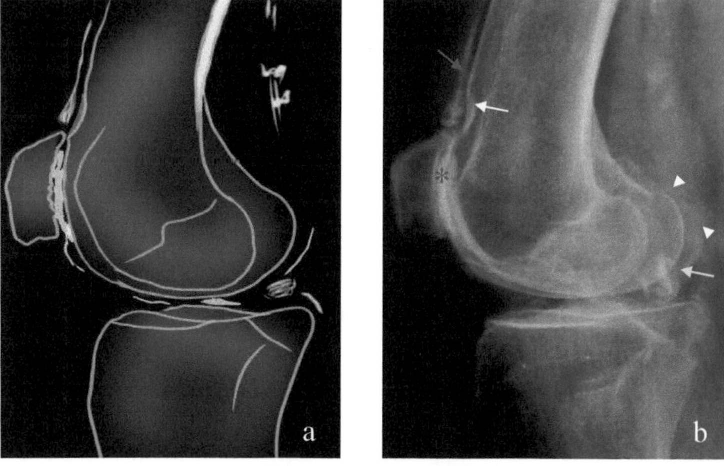

Fig. 59. Articular chondrocalcinosis. (a) Diagrams. (b) Profile X-ray of knee. Patellofemoral arthropathy (asterisk) with supratrochlear femoral erosion (white arrow), hyaline cartilage calcifications (arrowheads), meniscal calcification (yellow arrow) and quadriceps tendon calcifications (red arrow).

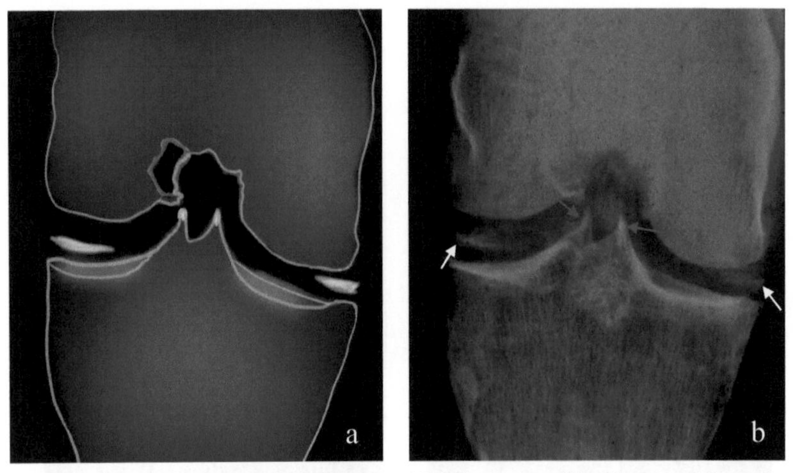

Fig. 60. Articular chondrocalcinosis. (a) Diagrams. (b) X-ray of front knee. Subchondral geodes (asterisk), opposite central osteophytes of the intercondylar notch (red arrow), meniscal calcification (white arrows).

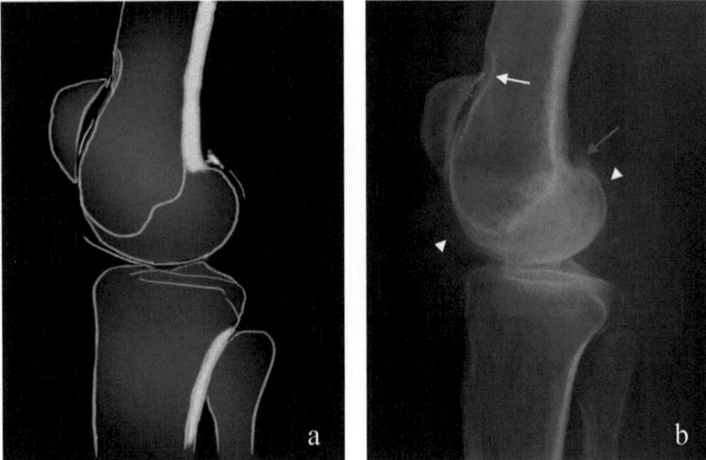

Fig. 61. Articular chondrocalcinosis. (a) Diagrams. (b) Profile X-ray of knee. Patellofemoral arthropathy (asterisk) with supratrochlear femoral erosion (white arrow), calcifications of hyaline cartilage (arrowheads) and calcifications of gastrocnemius tendons (red arrow).

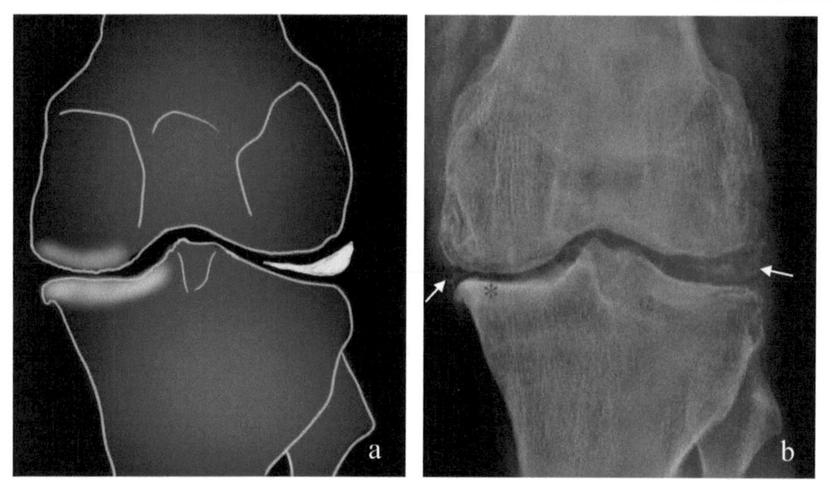

Fig. 62. Articular chondrocalcinosis. (a) Diagrams. (b) X-ray of the front knee. Alteration of tibial plateaus with misalignment (asterisk). Meniscal calcifications (white arrows).

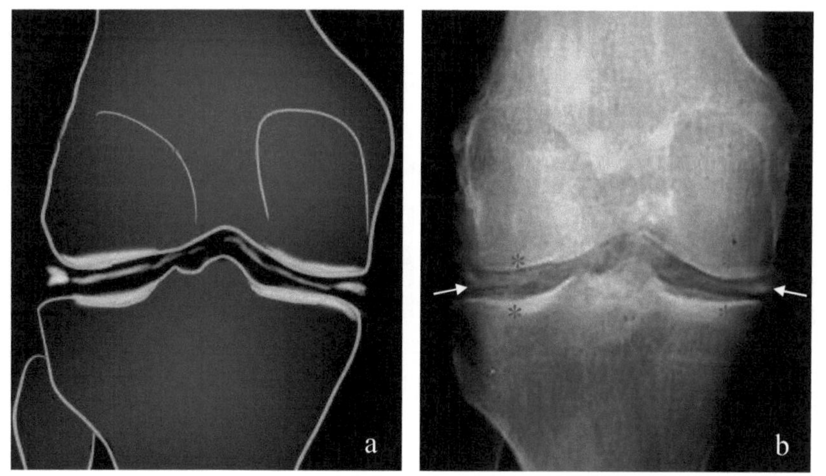

Fig. 63. Articular chondrocalcinosis. (a) Diagrams. (b) Frontal radiograph of knee. Meniscal calcifications, hyaline cartilage calcifications (arrows) and thin blades of subchondral osteosclerosis on either side of the joint (asterisks), giving the rail image.

1.1.2.2.Hands and wrists

Involvement often involves the lunopyramidal space and the triangular ligament of the carpus. These include :

- carpal bone cartilage calcifications (fig. 54, 64);
- calcifications of the triangular ligament of the carpus (fig. 54, 64);
- periarticular tendon calcifications, often in the metacarpophalangeal joints (fig. 65).

In chronic forms, destructive lesions can be seen:

- notches in the carpal bones;
- osteolysis mimicking arthritis;
- erosions of the lower end of the radius;
- trapeziometacarpal or radiocarpal pseudoarthropathy, often involving the radioscaphoid space [62] ;
- isolated involvement of the scaphotrapezial joint and the metacarpophalangeal joints of the 2eme and 3eme fingers are specific to the condition (fig. 66).

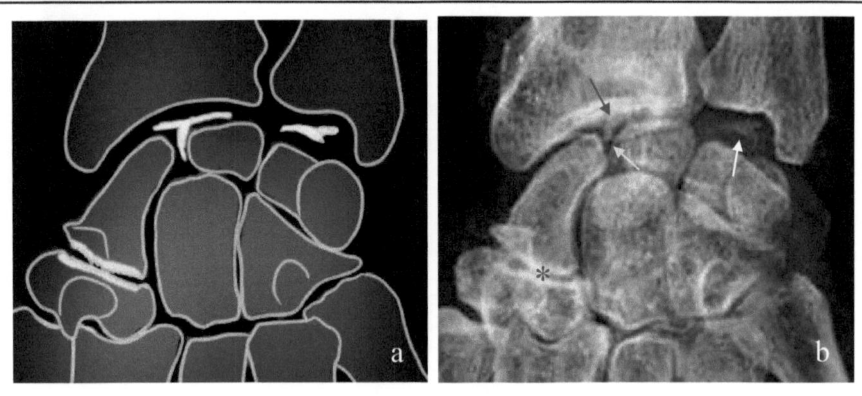

Fig. 64. Articular chondrocalcinosis. (a) Diagrams. (b) Front X-ray of the hand. Calcifications of the carpal triangular ligament (white arrow), hyaline cartilage (yellow arrows) and scapholunate and lunotriquetral ligaments (red arrows). Scaphotrapezial osteoarthritis (asterisk).

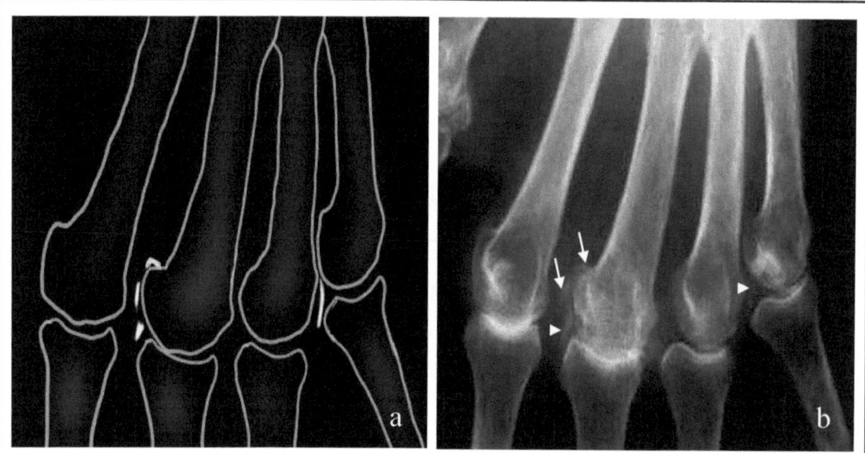

Fig. 65. Articular chondrocalcinosis. (a) Diagrams. (b) Facing radiograph of fingers. Tendon calcifications in the third metacarpophalangeal joint (arrows) and hyaline cartilage (arrowheads).

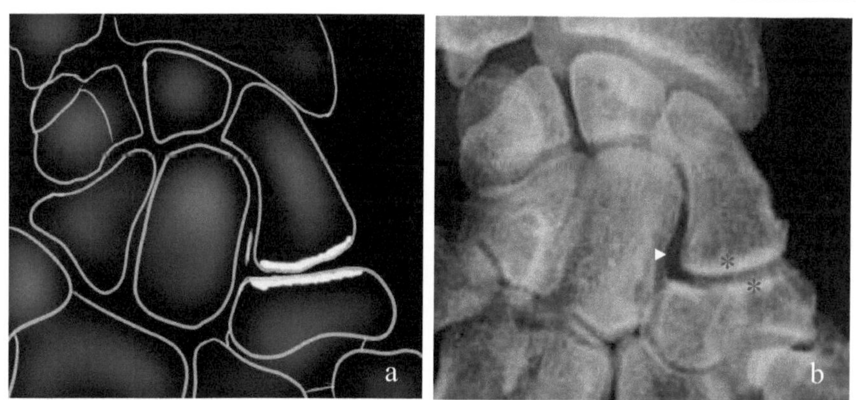

Fig. 66. Articular chondrocalcinosis. (a) Diagrams. (b) Front X-ray of the hand. Scaphotrapezial arthropathy with banded subchondral osteocondensation, indicating the severity of the arthropathy, even though joint pinching is not apparent in this view of the hand (asterisks). Calcification of hyaline cartilage (arrowhead).

1.1.2.3.Basin

Involvement is mainly found in the symphysis pubis and coxofemoral joint, and rarely in the sacroiliac joint.

Standard radiographs show calcifications:

- fibrocartilage of the symphysis pubis (fig. 53);
- cartilage crusting ;
- acetabular ribs and round ligaments (fig. 67);
- periarticular tendons (fig. 68);
- sacroiliac joints;

Destructive lesions may be observed at the symphysis (fig. 69) and at the coxofemoral joints.

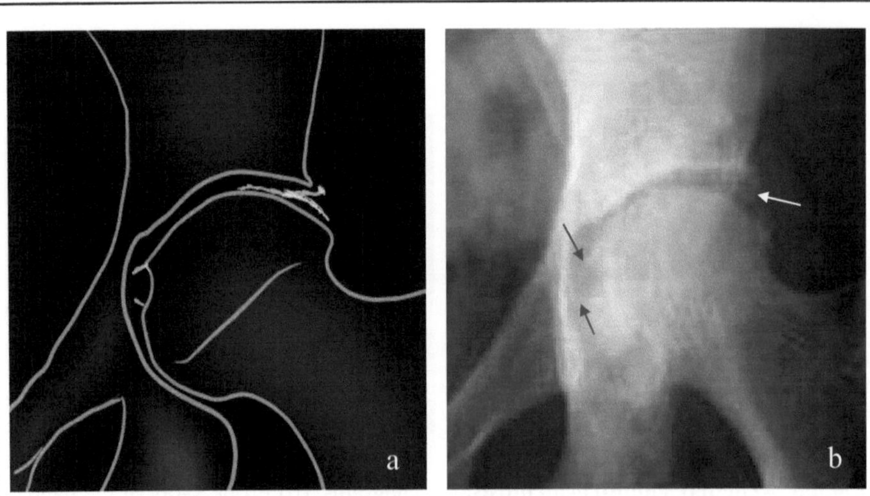

Fig. 67. Articular chondrocalcinosis. (a) Diagrams. (b) Front X-ray of the hip joint. Calcifications of acetabular bulges (white arrow) and round ligaments (red arrows).

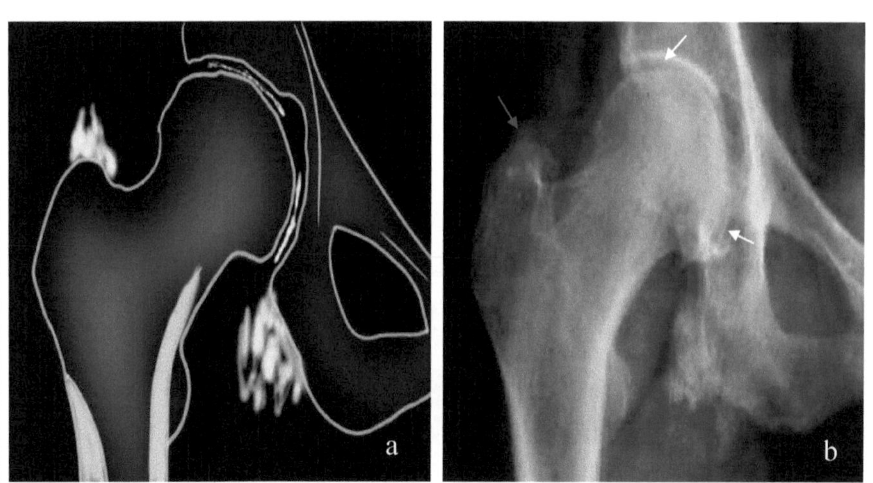

Fig. 68. Articular chondrocalcinosis. (a) Diagrams. (b) Front X-ray of the hip joint. Calcific border of the hip joint space (white arrows). Musculotendinous calcifications (red arrows).

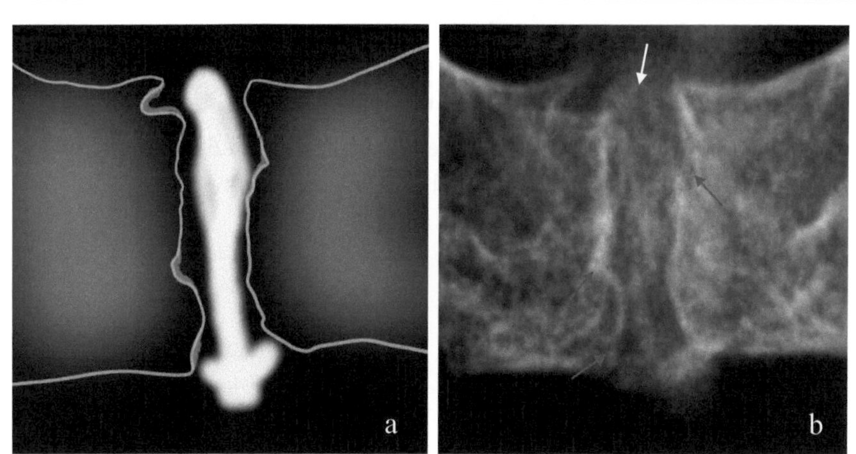

Fig. 69. Articular chondrocalcinosis. (a) Diagrams. (b) Frontal radiograph of pubic symphysis. Intracartilaginous opaque border of the pubic symphysis (white arrows). Subchondral erosions (red arrows).

1.1.2.4.Elbow

On standard films, capsulosynovial or tendinous calcifications are often seen in the triceps (fig. 70).

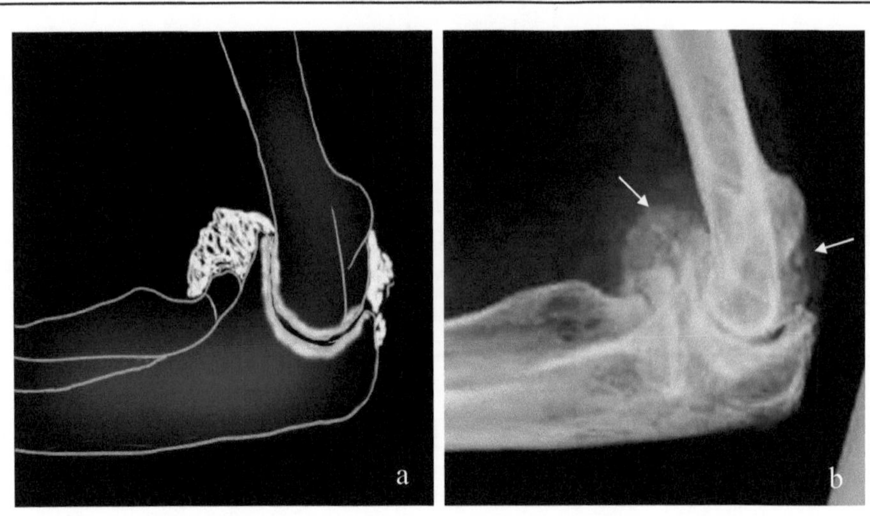

Fig. 70. Articular chondrocalcinosis. (a) Diagrams. (b) Profile X-ray of elbow. Elbow arthropathy with capsulo-synovial calcifications (arrows) [61].

1.1.2.5.Shoulder

Calcifications are mainly located in the cartilage of the humeral heads (Fig. 71), particularly in the superomedial region and at the acromioclavicular joints. Calcifications of the glenoid bulge, tendon calcifications of the supraspinatus, long biceps and subscapularis are best seen on CT.

In chronic forms, erosions of the humeral heads and articular surfaces can be seen on standard radiography [63].

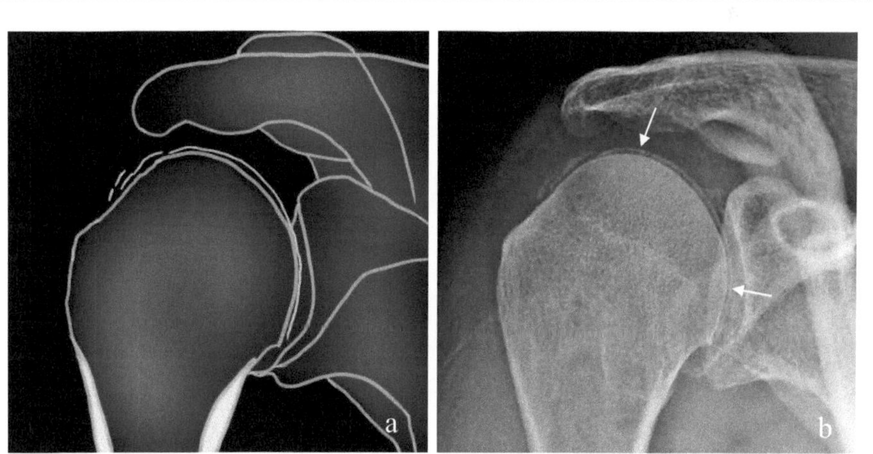

Fig. 71. Articular chondrocalcinosis. (a) Diagrams. (b) Front X-ray of shoulder. Calcifications of hyaline cartilage (arrows).

1.1.2.6.Spine

All floors may be affected, as well as the cervico-occipital hinge. Involvement predominates in the dorsolumbar region:

- calcification of the annulus fibrosus of the intervertebral discs (fig. 72, 73);
- calcium deposits in the vertebral endplates, transverse ligaments and yellow ligament (figs. 72, 73).

In chronic forms, destructive lesions give a pseudoarthrosic appearance with disc pinching and irregular sclerosis of the vertebral endplates (fig. 74).

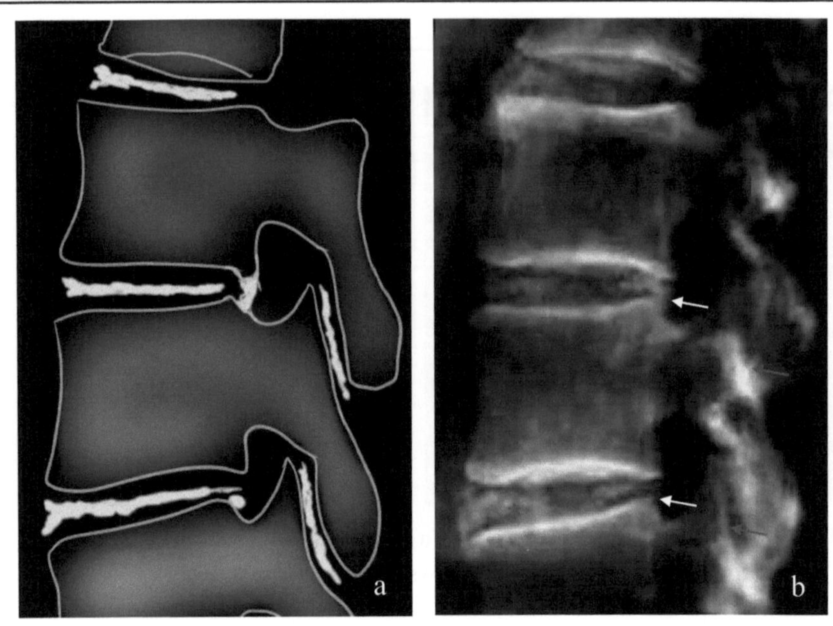

Fig. 72. Chondrocalcinosis (a) Diagrams. (b) Profile X-ray of lumbar spine. Calcification of the annulus fibrosus of the intervertebral discs (asterisks), yellow ligaments (white arrows). Posterior interapohyseal arthropathies associated with calcifications of the posterior interapohyseal joint spaces (red arrows).

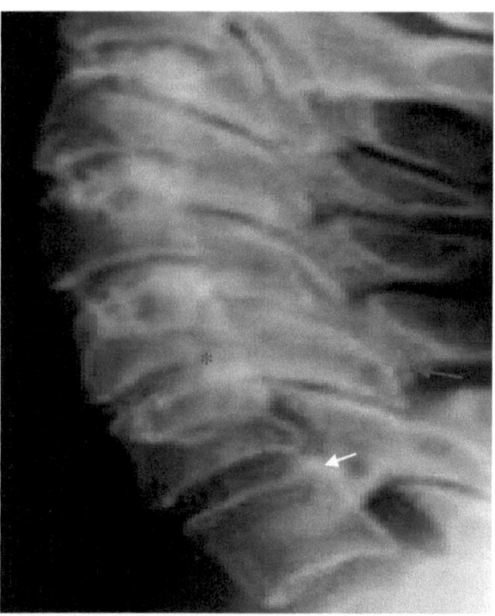

Fig. 73. Chondrocalcinosis. Radiograph of the cervical spine in profile. Calcification of the annulus fibrosus of the intervertebral discs (asterisks), yellow ligaments (white arrow) and posterior interapohyseal joint spaces (red arrows).

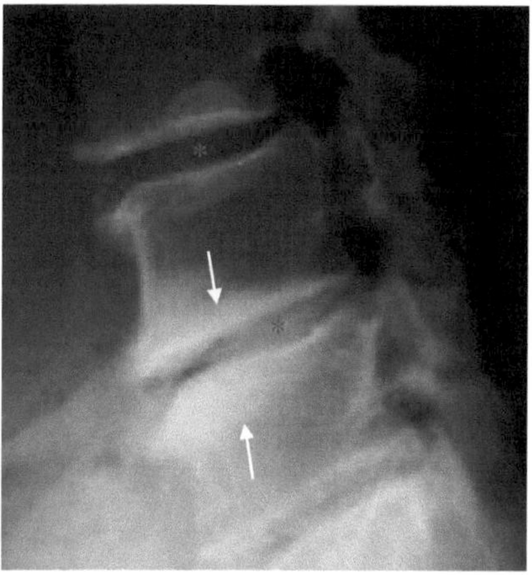

Fig. 74. Chondrocalcinosis. Lumbar spine radiograph in profile. Pseudoarthrosic appearance with disc pinching and irregular sclerosis of the vertebral endplates (arrows). Calcification of the annulus fibrosus of the intervertebral discs (asterisks) [64].

1.2. Ultrasound

Ultrasound will seek to identify calcium deposits in cartilage, fibrocartilage and tendons, as well as in synovial fluid.

1.2.1. Cartilage, fibrocartilage and tendon calcifications

These calcifications present as a hyperechoic line parallel to the cartilage surface and bone cortex, with no posterior acoustic effect due to their low density [65, 66]. (fig. 75). The most frequently affected locations accessible by ultrasound are, for cartilaginous deposits, the femoral condyles and metacarpal heads, and for fibrocartilaginous deposits, the triangular ligament of the carpus and the medial and lateral menisci of the knees (fig. 76). In some cases, hyperechoic deposits can also be found in tendons such as the Achilles tendon, or in bursae.

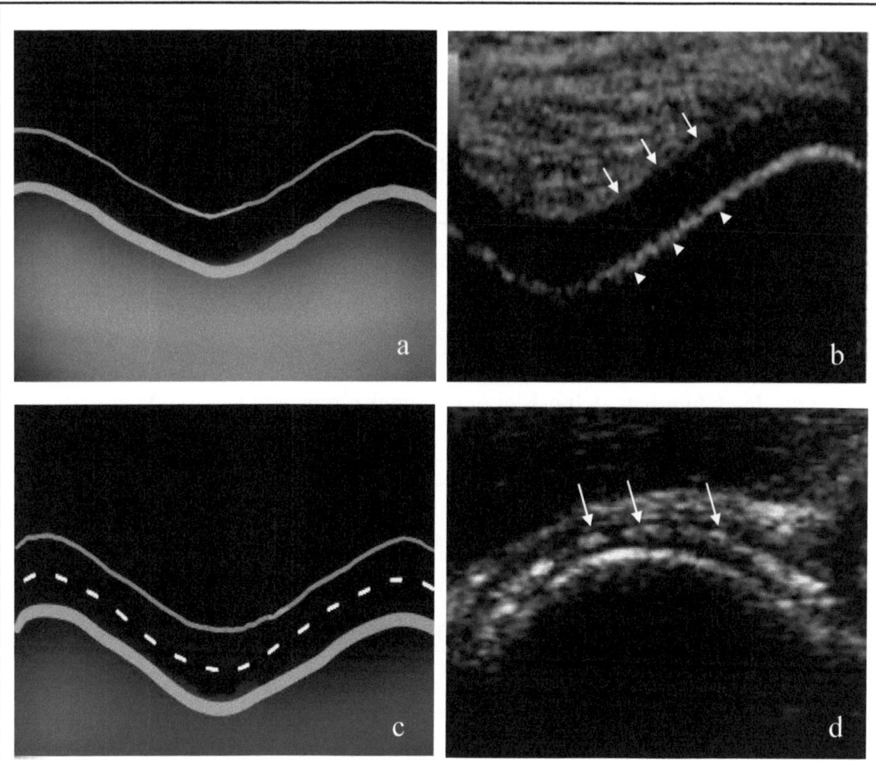

Fig. 75. Articular chondrocalcinosis. (a+c) Diagrams. (b+d) Ultrasound sections. (a+b). Normal anechogenic cartilage surface (arrows), cortical bone (arrowheads). (c+d) Discontinuous hyperechoic intra-cartilage band parallel to cartilage surface (arrows).

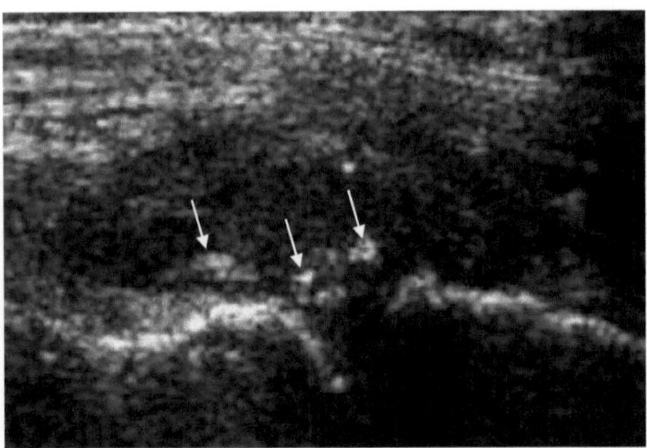

Fig. 76. Chondrocalcinosis. Longitudinal ultrasound section Meniscal calcifications (arrows) [45].

1.2.2. Hyperechoic calcifications in synovial fluid

They appear as floating hyperechoic joint spots, with rounded contours and sharp boundaries [65, 66]. The most frequently affected sites accessible by ultrasound are the quadricipital recesses and popliteal cysts (fig.77).

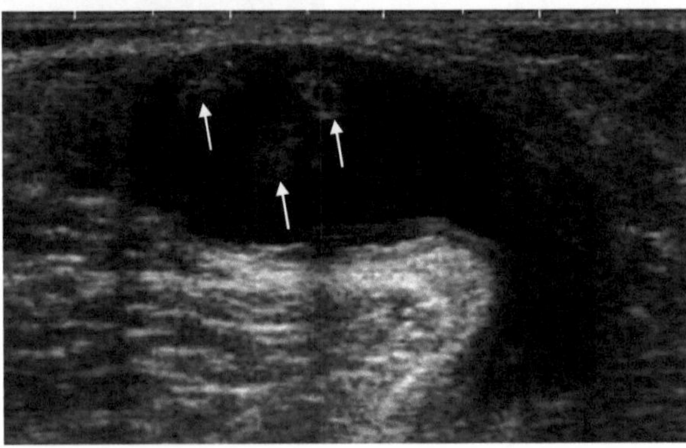

Fig. 77. Chondrocalcinosis. Longitudinal ultrasound section. Popliteal cyst shows hyperechoic images in its own right (arrows) [67].

Apatitic rheumatism

Apatitic rheumatism is related to deposits of apatite microcrystals, which may be secondary to elevated phosphocalcic product in cases of end-stage renal failure or vitamin D intoxication, but often no biological abnormality is found. Microcrystals are mainly deposited in tendons and periarticular bursae. The most common site is the supraspinatus tendon, where cloudy calcification is seen in 2-3% of the adult population [68]. The age of discovery is often between 40 and 60 in women, but can occur at any age [69]. Periarticular calcifications are often monoarticular, but may be polyarticular. Tendon calcifications are usually asymptomatic. However, they may manifest as acute pain, particularly in the "hyperalgesic shoulder", due to migration of calcifications into the subacromial deltoid bursa, causing abrupt onset, total functional impotence, fever, etc. [70]. Other hyperalgesic localizations are possible, such as small joints of the hands and feet, intervertebral discs and long neck muscles. Pain may progress to chronicity. Signs of acute arthritis have been observed, with apatite crystals difficult to detect due to their small size. Some destructive arthropathies of the shoulder (Milwaukee shoulder) are thought to be secondary to apatite microcrystals [71].

1. Imaging

1.1. Standard radiography

Standard radiology is the examination of choice for diagnosis, although some are only accessible by CT scan.

Visible calcifications are typically dense, structureless, rounded, homogeneous, ranging in size from a few millimetres to 1.5 cm on average, and in suggestive sites: the supraspinatus tendon, the para-acetabular and para-trochanteric regions, etc. (figs. 78, 79, 80). Calcifications become less dense radiologically during an acute attack, taking on a cloudy appearance before disappearing completely through liquefaction of the calcific material [72].

Tendon calcifications may migrate into a bursa. However, changes in size and shape, or even the disappearance of calcifications, is possible (fig. 81). Occasionally, calcifications are found at a distance from the joint, for example in the paradiaphyseal region along the humerus or femur, and may create cortical erosions. Unusual localizations have been described in the sub-occipital and latero-odontoid region, such as the now classic "crowned tooth" image [73].

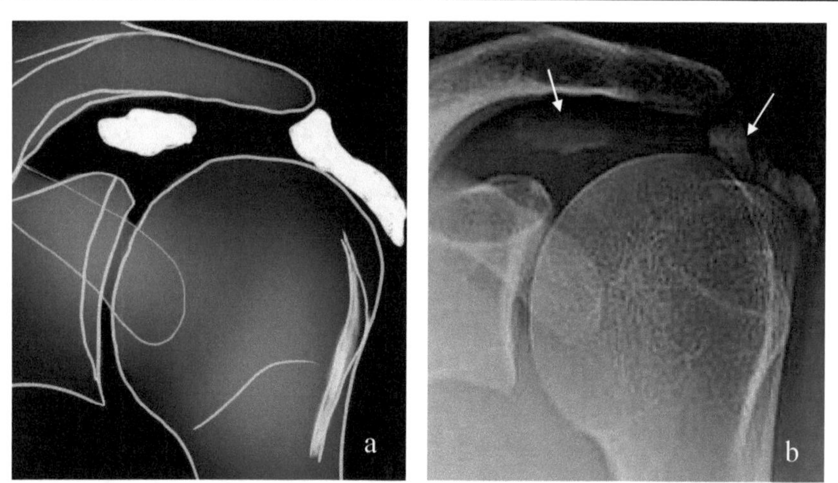

Fig. 78. Apatitic rheumatism (a) Diagrams. (b) Front X-ray of shoulder. Dense, structureless, homogeneous calcifications of varying size of the supraspinatus tendon (arrows) [74].

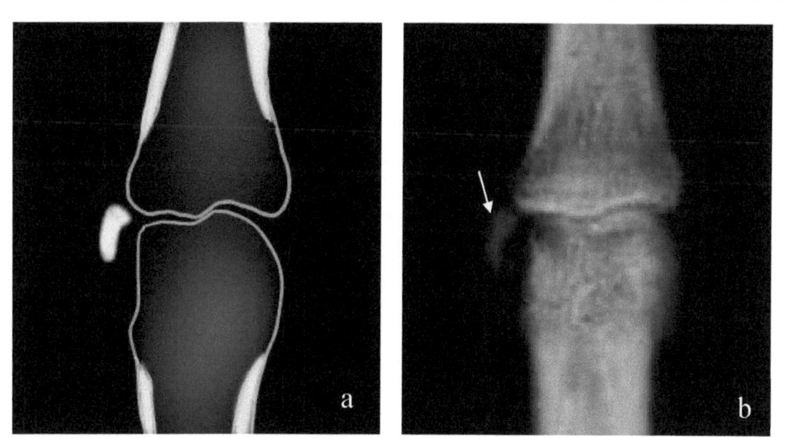

Fig. 79. Apatitic rheumatism (a) Diagrams. (b) Front X-ray of finger. Dense, homogeneous calcification of the para-articular tendon (arrow) [74].

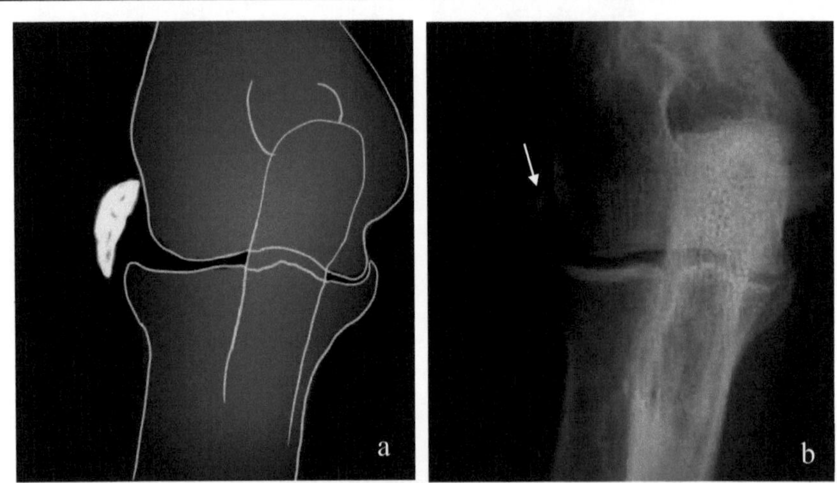

Fig. 80. Apatitic rheumatism (a) Diagrams. (b) Front X-ray of elbow. Para-articular tendon calcification (arrow) [74].

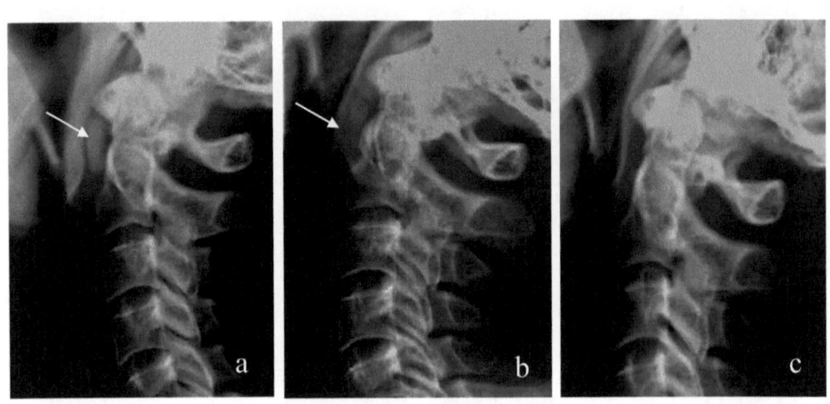

Fig. 81. Apatitic rheumatism. Radiograph of the spine in profile. (a) View on day 3. (b) View on day 15. (c) View after 3 months. Disappearance of tendon calcification in the long neck muscle (arrows) [74].

1.2. Ultrasound

Technical advances in ultrasonography, in particular its high spatial resolution and the hyperechoic nature of apatite microcrystals, have made this examination very interesting for diagnostic purposes [75] (fig. 82). Ultrasound allows precise localization of calcification and provides information on its consistency (soft or hard), enabling subsequent therapeutic management by puncture-aspiration [76]. Bone erosions at tendon insertion may be observed if the bone is superficial and accessible [77] (fig. 83).

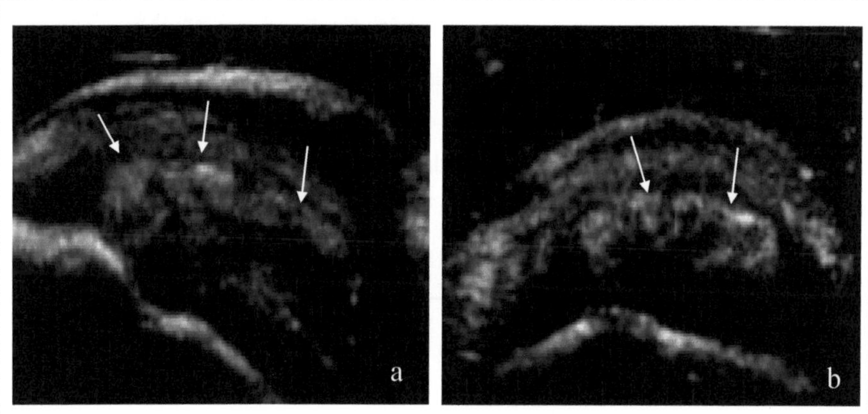

Fig. 82. Apatitic rheumatism. Ultrasonographic sections of the shoulder: (a) frontal section. (b) sagittal section. Hyperechoic tendon calcifications (arrows) [74].

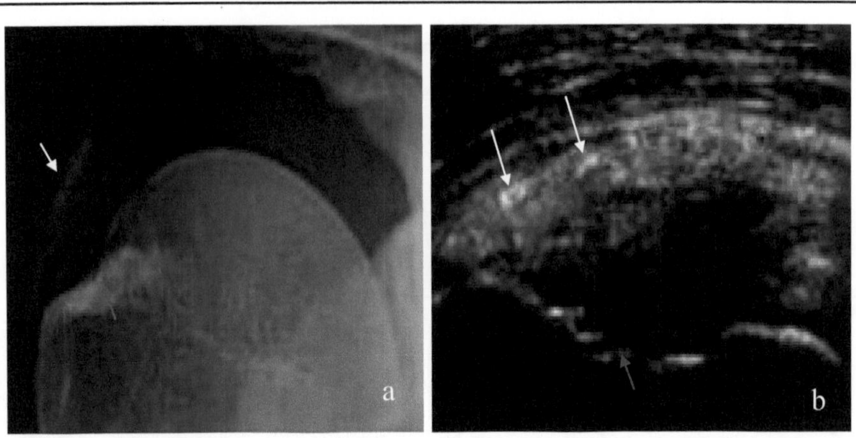

Fig. 83. Apatitic rheumatism. (a) Standard X-ray of the shoulder. (b) Ultrasound section of the shoulder. Tendon calcifications (white arrows) with bone erosion opposite (red arrows) [74].

1.3. Scanner

It is the examination of choice for unusual locations of calcific tendinopathy (fig. 84). In cases where calcifications have disappeared on radiographic films, CT scans can reveal a fine calcific line. This examination is also indicated in cases of unusual topography or particularly marked clinical or laboratory signs of inflammation. It remains the most efficient means of diagnosing periarticular and intra-articular calcifications.

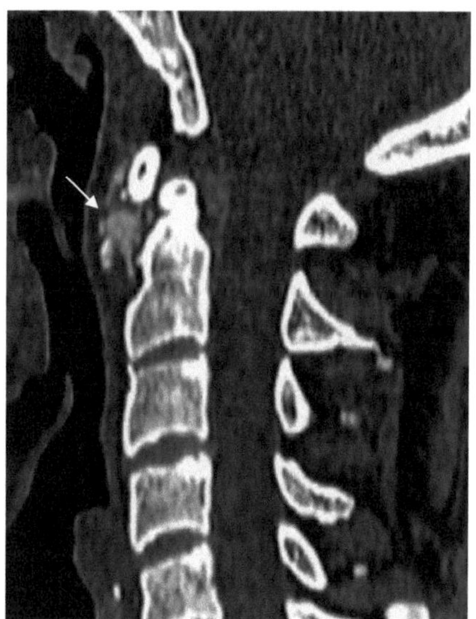

Fig. 84. Apatitic rheumatism. CT scan in sagittal reconstruction. Calcification of the tendon of the long neck muscle (arrow).

References

1. Richette P, Bardin T. Gout. Lancet 2010;375:318-28.
2. Dalbeth N, So A. Hyperuricemia and gout: state of the art and future perspectives. Ann Rheum Dis 2010;69:1737-43.
3. Neogi T. Gout. N Engl J Med 2011;364:443-52.
4. Ea HK. From hyperuric√©mia √† to gout: pathophysiology. Rev Rhum 2011;78(Suppl. 3):S103-8.
5. Wortmann RL. Gout and hyperuricemia. In: Kelley's textbook of Rheumatology. Philadelphia: Saunders Elsevier; 2009. p. 1481-506.
6. McLean L, Becker MA. Etiology and pathogeny of gout. In: Hochberg MA, Silman AJ, Smolen JS, Weinblatt ME, Weisman MH, editors. Rheumatology. London: Elsevier; 2011. p. 1841-57.
7. Yu TF. Some unusual features of gouty arthritis in females. Semin Arthritis Rheum 1977; 6: 247.
8. Yu TF. Diversity of clinical features in gouty arthritis. Semin Arthritis Rheum 1984; 13: 360-368.
9. Neogi T, Jansen TLTA, Dalbeth N, et al. 2015 Gout classification criteria: an American College of Rheumatology/European League Against Rheumatism collaborative initiative. Am Rheum Dis, 2015;74:1789-1798.
10. Fernandes EA, Bergamaschi SB, Rodrigues TC, Dias GC, Malmann R, Ramos GM, et al. Relevant aspects of imaging in the diagnosis and management of gout. Revista brasileira de reumatologia. 2016.
11. Egan R, Sartoris D, Resnick D. Radiographic features ofgout in the foot. J Foot Surg 1987; 26: 434-439.

12.Rettenbacher T, Ennemoser S, Weirich H, Ulmer H, Hartig F, Klotz W, et al. Diagnostic imaging of gout: comparison of high-resolution US versus conventional X-ray. Eur Radiol. 2008;18(3):621-30.

13.Cornelius R, Schneider H. Goutyarthritis in the adult. Radiol Clin North Am 1988; 26: 1267-1276.

14.Cortet B, Duquesnoy B, Amoura I, Bourgeois P, Delcambre B.Goutwith ankylosis. RevRhum(engl ed)1994;61: 44-47.

15.Cotten A. Imaging of os√©oarticular pathology. Practical s√©miology. In: Cotten A √©d. La goutte. Paris : Masson, 1998 : 24-26.

16.Martel W. The overhanging margin of bone: a roentgenologic manifestation of gout. Radiology 1968; 91: 755-756.

17.Resnick D, Niwayama G. Diagnosis of bone and joint disorders. In: Resnick D ed. Gouty arthritis. Philadelphia : WB Saunders, 1995 : 1511-1555.

18.Wright JT. Unusual manifestations of gout. Australas Radiol 1966; 10: 365.

19.Teh J, McQueen F, Eshed I, Advanced Imaging in the Diagnosis of Gout and Other Crystal Arthropathies. Semin Musculoskelet Radiol. 2018;22:225-236.

20.Cotten A, Boutry N, Demondion X, Delfaut E, Paul C, Chastanet P and Flipo RM. Goutte. Encycl M√©d Chir, Radiodiagnosis - Neuroradiology-Locomotor apparatus, 31-315-A-10, 2001, 10 p.

21.Cotton A, Pascart T and Corte B. Affections microcristallines. Medicine Key Fastest Medicine Insight Engine.

22.Gelberman RH, Doty DH, Hamer ML. Tophaceous gout involving the proximal interphalangeal joint. Clin Orthop, 1980; 147: 225-229.

23.Chiu KY, Leung F, Chow SP. Severe patellar destruction by infected chronic tophaceous gout. J Orthop Rheumatol, 1992; 5: 113.

24.Walot I, Staple TW. Case report 539. Skeletal Radiol, 1989; 18: 233.

25.Aaron SL, Miller JD, Percy JS. Tophaceous gout in the cervical spine. J Rheumatol, 1984; 11: 862-865.

26.Arnold MH, Brooks PM, Savvas P, Ruff S. Tophaceous gout of the axial skeleton. Aust NZ J Med, 1988; 18: 865-867.

27.Clerc D, Marfeuille M, Labous E, Desmoulins F, Quillard J, Bisson M. Spinal tophaceous gout. Clin Exp Rheumatol, 1998 ; 16 : 621.

28.Fenton P, Young S, Prutis K. Gout of the spine: two case reports and a review of the literature. J Bone Joint Surg Am, 1995; 77: 767-771.

29.Miller LJ, Pruett SW, Losada R, Fruauff A, Sagerman P. Tophaceous gout of the lumbar spine: MR findings. J Comput Assist Tomogr, 1996; 20: 1004-1005.

30.Staub-Schmidt T, Chaouat A, Rey D, Bloch JG, Christmann D. Spinal involvement in gout. Arthritis Rheum, 1995 ; 38 : 139-141.

31.Vervaeck M, De Keyser J, Pauwels P, Frecourt N, D'Haens J, Ebinger G. Sudden hypotonic paraparesis caused by tophaceous gout of the lumbar spine. Clin Neurol Neurosurg, 1991 ; 93 : 233-236.

32.Ottaviani S, Bardin T and Richette P: Usefulness of ultrasonography for gout. Joint Bone Spine 2012, 79:441-5.

33.Perez-Ruiz F, Dalbeth N, Urresola A, et al: Gout. Imaging of gout: findings and utility. Arthritis Res Ther 2009, 11:232.

34.Filippucci E, Scire CA, Delle Sedie A, et al: Ultrasound imaging for the rheumatologist. XXV. Sonographic assessment of the knee in patients with gout and calcium pyrophosphate deposition disease. Clin Exp Rheumatol 2010, 28:2-5.

35.Wakefield RJ, Balint PV, Szkudlarek M, et al; OMERACT 7 Special Interest Group.Musculoskeletal ultrasound including definitions for ultrasonographic pathology. J Rheumatol, 2005;32(12):2485-2487.

36.Rettenbacher T, Ennemoser S, Weirich H, et al: Diagnostic imaging of gout: comparison of high-resolution US versus conventional X-ray. Eur Radiol 2008, 18:621-30.

37.Ottaviani S, Bardin T and Richette P. Int√©r√™t of √©chography in gout. Revue du Rhumatisme, 2012, 79(4), 301-305.

38.Ottaviani S, Allard A, Bardin T, et al: Ultrasonography findings in early gout. Clin Exp Rheumatol 2011, 29:816-21.

39.Ottaviani S, Richette P, Allard A, et al: Ultrasonography in gout: a case-control study. Clin Exp Rheumatol 2012, 30:499-504.

40.Terslev L, Gutierrez M, Christensen R, et al; OMERACT US Gout Task Force. Assessing elementary lesions in gout by ultrasound:results of an OMERACT patient-based agreement and reliability exercise. J Rheumatol 2015;42(11):2149-2154.

41.Gutierrez M, Schmidt WA, Thiele RG, et al; OMERACT Ultrasound Gout Task Force group. International Consensus for ultrasound lesions in gout: results of Delphi process and web-reliability exercise. Rheumatology (Oxford) 2015;54(10):1797-1805.

42.Min, H. K., Cho, H., & Park, H. Pilot study: Asymptomatic hyperuricemia patients with obesity and nonalcoholic fatty liver disease have increased risk of double contour sign. The Korean Journal of Internal Medicine, 2020, 35(6), 1517-1523.

43.Ottaviani S. Ultrasonography in gout. Rhum Afr Franc 2020; 3 (1): 1 - 7.

44.Cotten A, Pascart T, Cortet B. Microcrystalline affections. Imagerie musculosquelettique - Pathologies g√©n√©rales, 2e √©dition 2013, Elsevier Masson SAS.

45.Ottaviani S. √achography in microcrystalline arthropathies. Revue du Rhumatisme Monographies, 2015, 82(4), 181-186.

46.Omoumi P, Becce F, Racine D, Ott JG, Andreisek G, Verdun FR. Dual-Energy CT: basic principles, technical approaches, and applications in musculoskeletal imaging (Part 1). Semin Musculoskelet Radiol 2015;19(5):431-7.

47.McQueen FM, Doyle A, Dalbeth N. Imaging in gout-what can we learn from MRI, CT, DECT and US? Arthritis Res Therapy 2011;13(6):246.

48.Bongartz T, Glazebrook KN, Kavros SJ, Murthy NS, Merry SP, Franz 3rd WB, et al. Dual-energy CT for the diagnosis of gout: an accuracy and diagnostic yield study. Ann Rheum Dis 2015;74(6):1072-7.

49.Melzer R, Pauli C, Treumann T, Krauss B. Gout tophis detection-a comparison of dual-energy CT (DECT) and histology. Semin Arthritis Rheum 2014;43 (5):662-5.

50.Durcan L, Grainger R, Keen HI, Taylor WJ, Dalbeth N. Imaging as a potential outcome measure in gout studies: A systematic literature review. Semin Arthritis Rheum 2016;45(5):570-9.

51.Teh J, McQueen F, Eshed I, Advanced Imaging in the Diagnosis of Gout and Other Crystal Arthropathies. Semin Musculoskelet Radiol 2018; 22:225-236.

52.Chowalloor PV, Siew TK, Keen HI. Imaging in gout: A review of the recent developments. Therap Adv Musculoskelet Dis 2014;6(4):131-43.

53.Reginato AJ, Tamesis E, Netter P. Familial and clinical aspects of calcium pyrophosphate deposition disease. Curr Rheumatol Rep 1999 ; 1 : 112-120.

54.Delauche MC, Stehle B, Verret JM, Kahn MF, Cassou B. Frequency of radiological chondrocalcinosis after age 80. A prospective study. RevRhumMalOstéoartic1977;44: 555-557.

55.Mitrovic D, Stankovic A, Morin J, Borda-Iriarte O, Uzan M, Quintero M et al. Anatomical frequency of meniscochondrocalcinosis of the knee. Rev Rhum Mal Ostéoartic 1982; 49: 495-499.

56.Wilkins E, Dieppe P, Maddison P, Evinson G. Osteoarthritis and articular chondrocalcinosis in the elderly. Ann Rheum Dis 1983; 42: 280-284.

57.Menkes CJ, Simon F, Choukari L, Ecoffet M, Amor B, Delbarre F. The destructive arthropathies of chondrocalcinosis. Rev Rhum Mal Ostéoartic 1973; 40: 115-123.

58.Villiaumey J, Larget-Piet B, Di Menza C, Rotterdam M. Symptomatic and evolutionary features of joint destruction observed during chondrocalcinosis. Rev Rhum Mal Ostéoartic 1975; 42: 263-273.

59.Foldes K, Lenchik L, Jaovisidha S, Clopton P, Sartoris DJ, Resnick D. Association of gastrocnemius tendon calcification with chondrocalcinosis of the knee. Skeletal Radiol 1996; 25: 621-624.

60.Yang BY, Sartoris DJ, Resnick D, Clopton P. Calcium pyrophosphate dihydrate crystal deposition disease: frequency of tendon calcification about the knee. J Rheumatol 1996; 23: 883-888.

61.Deries B, Delfaut E, Cortet B, Boutry N, Paul C and Cotten A. Arthropathies with microcrystals (except uratic and calcium hydroxyapatite crystals). Encycl Méd Chir, Radiodiagnostic - Neuroradiologie-Appareil locomoteur, 31-316-A-10, 2002, 13 p.

62.Donich AS, Lektrakul N, Liu CC, Theodorou DJ, Kakitsubata Y, Resnick D. Calcium pyrophosphate dihydrate crystal deposition disease of the wrist: trapezioscaphoid joint abnormality. J Rheumatol 2000; 27: 2628-2634.

63.Resnick D, Niwayama G. Calcium pyrophosphate dihydrate (CPPD) crystal deposition disease. In: Resnick D ed. Hemochromatosis and Wilson's disease. Diagnosis of bone and joint disorders. Philadelphia : WB Saunders, 1995 : 1556-1614.

64.Benoist M., & Polack Y. Spinal manifestations of articular chondrocalcinosis. Revue du Rhumatisme, 2007, 74(2), 188-193.

65. FoltzV, Gandjbakhch F, Etchepare F, Rosenberg C, Tanguy ML, Rozenberg S, et al. Power Doppler ultrasound, but not low-field magnetic resonance imaging, predicts relapse and radiographic disease progression in rheumatoid arthritis patients with low levels of disease activity. Arthritis Rheum;64(1):67-76.
66. Scire CA, Montecucco C, Codullo V, Epis O, Todoerti M, Caporali R. Ultrasonographic evaluation of joint involvement in early rheumatoid arthritis in clinical remission: power Doppler signal predicts short-term relapse. Rheumatology (Oxford) 2009;48(9):1092-7.
67. Banal F. Ultrasound semiology in inflammatory and microcrystalline rheumatism. Revue Réflexions rhumatologiques, 2012, 149, tome 16.
68. Amor B, Cherot A, Delbarre F. Hydroxyapatite rheumatism (multiple tendon calcification disease). I- étude clinique. Rev Rhum Mal Osteoartic 1977;44:301-8.
69. Halverson PB. Crystal deposition disease of the shoulder (including calcific tendinoitis and Milwaukee shoulder syndrome). Curr Rheumatol Rep 2003;5:244-7.
70. Hamada J, Tamai K, Ono W, Saotome K. Does the nature of deposited basic calcium phosphate crystals determine clinical course in calcific periarthritis of the shoulder? J Rheumatol 2006;33:326-32.
71. McCarty DJ, Halverson PB, Carrera GF. "Milwaukee shoulder": association of microspheroids containing hydroxyapatite crystals, active collagenase, and neutral protease with rotator cuff defects. Arthritis Rheum 1981;24:464-73.
72. Fritz P, Bardin T, Laredo JD, Ziza JM, D'Anlejan G, Lansaman J, et al. Paradiaphyseal calcific tendinitis with cortical bone erosion. Arthritis Rheum 1994;37:718-23.
73. Alcalay M, Ferrier N, Vandermarcq P, Le Goff P, Le Parc JP, Bontoux D. Crowned odontoid syndrome. A propos de 4 cas. In: Gaucher A, Netter P, Pourel J, Régent D, editors. Actualités en physiologie et pharmacologie articulaires. Paris: Masson; 1991. p. 99-106.

74.http://onclepaul.fr/wp-content/uploads/2011/07/localisationsrachidiennes-et-cervicales-du-rhumatisme-à-apatite.pdf.
75.Wiener SN, Seitz Jr WH. Sonography of the shoulder in patients with tears of the rotator cuff: accuracy and value for selecting surgical options. AJR Am J Roentgenol 1993;160:103-7.
76.Lecoq B, Levasseur R, Fournier L, Schmutz G, Marcelli C. Atypical pattern of acute severe shoulder pain: contribution of sonography. Joint Bone Spine 2004;71:592-4.
77.Garcia GM, McCord GC, Kumar R. Hydroxyapatite crystal deposition disease. Semin Musculoskelet Radiol 2003;7:187-93.

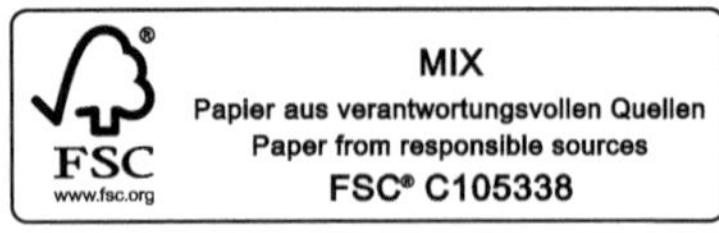

Printed by Books on Demand GmbH, Norderstedt / Germany